Ultrasound Essentials

A REFERENCE GUIDE TO NORMAL ANATOMY AND EXAM PROTOCOLS FOR THE EMERGING SONOGRAPHER

Lexie Skordahl, RDMS, RVT

Please know that these values have been gathered from current literature on the market. Know that these values can change over time as medicine becomes better and better. Also, know that individual departments can also use their own set of values and they may not match exactly to the values provided in this guide.

All of the ultrasound images in this book are taken of volunteers. NONE of the images are taken of patients, nor did I ask any of the patients to volunteer. The volunteers are people who I know personally that wanted to help me with my book.

Paperback ISBN: 978-1-961429-03-1

E-Book ISBN: 978-1-961429-04-8

Library of Congress Control Number: 2025918569

1st Edition 2024

Cover Art By: GetCovers

Backwoods Books LLC

7202 NE Highway 99 STE 106 PMB 410,

Vancouver WA 98665

To students and fellow sonographers.

United as one, we make a fantastic team.

Contents

Introduction

Howdy! I'm excited that you have my book in your hands! My goal for this guide is to provide you with normal measurements and blood flow velocities of organs and vasculature. Keep in mind that these values are taken from current literature on the market as well as values that are used at my prior and current hospitals and clinics. Know that these values can vary from facility to facility. Feel free to write in your own measurements if you use something different than what is written in this guide. Also, feel free to reach out to me and let me know what your site uses if it differs from what is in my guide. I would be very interested to hear what is your normal! My email is in the back of the book.

Before we begin, I want to tell you a little bit about myself. I am a registered ARDMS sonographer and hold credentials in abdomen, obstetrics/gynecology, vascular, and breast. I attended a college in Northern Washington for my sonography program and completed my clinical internships at a large hospital in Bellevue, WA, and at a clinic in Vancouver, WA. Aside from my internships, I have worked at two hospitals and three clinics, so I know the ins and outs of both. I am currently working at a hospital/clinic, and I split my week between the two locations.

I hope that this guide provides easy, fast, and straightforward access to answers. We have so much information that we have to retain, that it can be difficult at times to remember every single normal measurement or every single blood flow velocity. This is why I created this guide! Use it to study for board exams or use it as a reference tool whenever needed. Let's get started!

I hope you enjoy!

~Lexie

Disclaimers

Measurements

Every department will use relatively similar measurement values. There may be some slight variation in measurements and I have tried to include those when necessary.

Protocols

Every sonographer and department will have their own way of scanning. The protocols listed in each chapter are sample protocols. You may use the protocols that I have provided or use the protocols that your clinical instructors, fellow sonographers, or department use.

Images

All of the ultrasound images in this book are taken of volunteer models. NONE of the images are taken of patients, nor did I ask any of the patients to volunteer.

Key

L: Length	P: Proximal	Sup: Superior	MED: Medial
AP: Anteroposterior	M: Mid	Inf: Inferior	ML: Midline
W: Width	D: Distal	M - L: Medial - Lateral	LAT: Lateral
SAG: Sagittal	RAD: Radial	RT: Right	BIF: Bifurcation
TRV: Transverse	ARAD: Antiradial	LT: Left	TT: Temporal Tap

Abbreviations + Acronyms

- 3VC: 3-Vessel Cord
- 3VT: 3-Vessel Trachea
- 3VTV: 3-Vessel Trachea View
- 3VV: 3-Vessel View
- 4-CH HRT: 4-Chamber Heart
- AAA: Abdominal Aortic Aneurysm
- AB: Abortion
- AB / ABD: Abdomen
- ABI: Ankle Brachial Index
- AC: Abdominal Circumference
- ACI: Abdominal Cord Insertion
- ADN: Adnexa

- AFI: Amniotic Fluid Index
- AFP: Alpha-fetoprotein
- ALP: Alkaline Phosphatase
- ALT: Alanine Aminotransferase
- AMA: Advanced Maternal Age / Against Medical Advice
- Ant: Anterior
- AO: Aorta
- AOA: Aortic Arch
- AOC: Area of Concern
- AP: Anteroposterior
- APPY: Appendix
- ARAD / ANTI-RAD: Antiradial
- ARDMS: American Registry of Diagnostic Medical Sonography
- ARFI: Acoustic Radiation Force Impulse
- AST: Aspartate Aminotransferase
- AT: Acceleration Time
- ATA: Anterior Tibial Artery
- AUB: Abnormal Uterine Bleeding

- AX: Axilla
- BE: Blind End
- BI-RADS: Breast Imaging Reporting and Data System
- BICAV: Bicaval
- BL: Bladder
- BMI: Body Mass Index
- BPD: Biparietal Diameter
- bpm: Beats Per Minute
- BPP: Biophysical Profile
- BR: Breast
- BRACH: Brachial
- BUN: Blood Urea Nitrogen
- Ca: Cancer
- CA: Celiac Artery
- CAD: Coronary Artery Disease
- CBD: Common Bile Duct
- CCA: Common Carotid Artery
- CDS: Cul-de-sac

- CFA: Common Femoral Artery
- CFV: Common Femoral Vein
- CHA: Common Hepatic Artery
- CIA: Common Iliac Artery
- CL: Corpus Luteum
- CMFN: Centimeters from Nipple
- CRL: Crown Rump Length
- CSF: Cerebrospinal Fluid
- CSP: Cavum Septum Pellucidum
- Cx: Canceled
- CX: Cervix
- DA: Ductal Arch
- D&C: Dilation and Curettage
- DP: Dorsalis Pedis
- DVT: Deep Venous Thrombosis
- ECA: External Carotid Artery
- ED: End Diastolic
- EDV: End Diastolic Velocity

- EIA: External Iliac Artery
- ENDO: Endometrium
- EPI: Epididymis
- Epi: Epigastric
- ETOH: Alcohol
- FBM: Fetal Breathing Movements
- FF: Free Fluid
- FHR: Fetal Heart Rate
- FL: Femur Length
- FP: Fetal Pole
- FV / SFV: Femoral Vein / Superficial Femoral Vein
- GA: Gestational Age
- GB: Gallbladder
- GFR: Glomerular Filtration Rate
- GS: Gestational Sac
- GSV: Great / Greater Saphenous Vein
- GYN: Gynecology
- HC: Head Circumference

- hCG: Human Chorionic Gonadotropin
- Hep: Hepatitis
- HRT: Hormone Replacement Therapy
- HTN: Hypertension
- HV: Hepatic Vein
- Hx: History
- IAC: Intersocietal Accreditation Commission
- IBS: Irritable Bowel Syndrome
- ICA: Internal Carotid Artery
- IIA: Internal Iliac Artery
- IMA: Inferior Mesenteric Artery
- IMT: Intima-Media Thickness
- Inf: Inferior
- IP: Inpatient
- IQR/M: Interquartile Range / Median
- Isth: Isthmus
- IUD: Intrauterine Device
- IVC: Inferior Vena Cava

- L: Length
- Lat: Lateral
- LDH: Lactic Dehydrogenase
- LE: Lower Extremity
- LEA: Lower Extremity Arterial
- LEV: Lower Extremity Venous
- LFT: Liver Function Test
- LHV: Left Hepatic Vein
- Liv: Liver
- LK: Left Kidney
- LLD: Left Lateral Decubitus
- LLQ: Left Lower Quadrant
- LN: Lymph Node
- LO / LT O: Left Ovary
- LPV: Left Portal Vein
- LRA: Left Renal Artery
- LRV: Left Renal Vein
- LUQ: Left Upper Quadrant

- LVOT: Left Ventricular Outflow Tract
- Mammo: Mammogram
- Med: Medial
- METAVIR: Meta-analysis of histological data in viral hepatitis
- MHV: Middle Hepatic Vein
- Mid: Middle
- MFM: Maternal Fetal Medicine
- MPV: Main Portal Vein
- MRI: Magnetic Resonance Imaging
- MVP: Maximum Vertical Pocket
- N / NIP: Nipple
- NB: Nasal Bone
- NICU: Neonatal Intensive Care Unit
- NPO: Nil Per Os "nothing by mouth"
- OB: Obstetrics
- OP: Outpatient
- PAD: Peripheral Artery Disease
- Palp: Palpable

- Panc: Pancreas
- PBH: Patient Body Habitus
- PCI: Placental Cord Insertion
- PE: Pulmonary Embolism
- PERO: Peroneal
- PF: Posterior Fossa
- PFA: Profunda Femoris Artery
- PFV: Profunda Femoris Vein
- PHTN: Portal Hypertension
- PI: Pulsatility Index
- Plac: Placenta
- PMB: Post-menopausal Bleeding
- PO: Per Os "by mouth"
- POP: Popliteal
- POS: Position
- Post: Posterior
- POST-MENO: Post-menopausal
- Prost: Prostate

- PS: Peak Systolic
- Pt: Patient
- PTA: Posterior Tibial Artery
- PTH: Parathyroid Hormone
- PV: Portal Vein
- Px: Pain
- RA: Retroareolar or Renal Artery
- Rad: Radiologist
- RAD: Radial
- RAR: Renal Aortic Ratio
- RAS: Renal Artery Stenosis
- RHV: Right Hepatic Vein
- RI: Resistive Index
- RK: Right Kidney
- RLD: Right Lateral Decubitus
- RLQ: Right Lower Quadrant
- RO / RT O: Right Ovary
- RPV: Right Portal Vein

- RRA: Right Renal Artery
- RRV: Right Renal Vein
- RUQ: Right Upper Quadrant
- RVOT: Right Ventricular Outflow Tract
- SA: Splenic Artery
- SAG: Sagittal
- SBCLV: Subclavian
- S/D: Systolic / Diastolic Ratio
- SFA: Superficial Femoral Artery
- SMA: Superior Mesenteric Artery
- SOB: Shortness of Breath
- SPL: Spleen
- Stom: Stomach
- SUBMAND: Submandibular
- Sup: Superior
- SV: Soleal Vein
- SVC: Superior Vena Cava
- T3: Triiodothyronine

- T4: Thyroxine
- TA: Transabdominal
- TEST: Testicle or Testosterone
- THY: Thyroid
- TI-RADS: Thyroid Imaging Reporting and Data System
- TIPS: Trans-jugular Intrahepatic Portosystemic Shunt
- TRV / Trans: Transverse
- TSH: Thyroid-stimulating Hormone
- TT: Temporal Tap
- TV: Transvaginal
- UE: Upper Extremity
- UEA: Upper Extremity Arterial
- UEV: Upper Extremity Venous
- ULN: Ulnar
- US: Ultrasound
- UT: Uterus
- UVJ: Ureterovesical Junction
- VB: Vaginal Bleeding

- VERT: Vertebral
- W: Width
- WBC: White Blood Cell
- WNL: Within Normal Limits

1

Abdomen

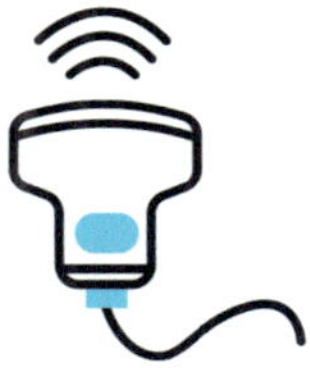

Abdomen Complete

Patient Prep and Exam

The patient needs to be NPO (nothing to eat or drink by mouth) for 8 hours prior to their exam. Eating and drinking causes bowel gas, obscuring the image quality of the organs and vessels.

Transducers Used

- Curvilinear C1-6

Exam Indications

- RUQ px
- Epi px
- Flank px
- Nausea/vomiting
- Elevated LFTs or other labs
- ETOH
- Bloating/abdominal distention

Functions and Labs

Structure:	Function:	Labs:
Aorta	The largest artery in the body that provides blood to all the extremities, organs, and tissues from the heart	Hematocrit
Appendix	A reservoir for healthy bacteria, that is released to help get rid of disease-causing organisms in the intestine	WBC
Common Bile Duct	Receives bile from the cystic duct. It then connects to the pancreatic duct. It carries bile down to the intestines to help aid digestion	Bilirubin
Gallbladder	A reservoir that holds bile. After food (containing fat) is consumed, the GB contracts, releasing bile to the CBD that then gets released to the duodenum to aid in digestion of those fats	Bilirubin
Inferior Vena Cava	The largest vein in the body that retrieves blood from all the extremities, organs, and tissues and brings that blood to the heart	
Hepatic Veins	They drain oxygen poor blood from the liver and into the IVC	
Kidneys	They filter blood, removing waste products through the form of urine They also maintain homeostasis and secrete hormones	BUN Creatinine GFR

Functions and Labs Continued

Structure:	Function:	Labs:
Liver	Produces bile, cholesterol, and proteins Converts glucose to glycogen Stores iron Converts ammonia to urea Filters poisonous substances out of the blood	Albumin ALP ALT AST
Main Portal Vein	Carries blood from the spleen and GI tract to the liver to be metabolized and detoxed	
Pancreas	Produces enzymes that help aid digestion Creates hormones, such as insulin, which lower blood sugar – and glucagon, which raises blood sugar	ALP Amylase Glucose Lipase
Spleen	Produces white blood cells Stores and filters blood	Hematocrit WBC

Helpful Tips

Take into consideration when determining what is "normal" for patients; for instance, organs tend to be on the larger side when the patient is tall. When patients are shorter, their organs tend to be smaller. For example, patients that are 5'3" shouldn't typically have kidneys measuring 13cm, and be considered "normal". Just like a pt (patient) who is 6'4", shouldn't have kidneys measuring 9cm. It CAN happen, but typically the organ size should reflect the patient's overall height.

<u>Pancreas:</u>

The pancreas is not normally something that is measured. In my 5+ years of scanning at multiple facilities, including an additional 2 years of my time in clinical internship, I have never measured a pancreas. I do, however, measure the Duct of Wirsung (also called the common pancreatic duct), if I can see it.

But never say never! You may find yourself at a location that does measure parts of the pancreas. Therefore, I have provided the measurements for you just in case.

Pancreas

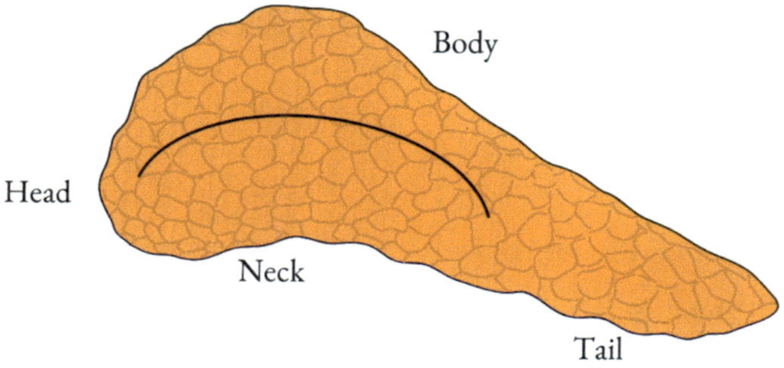

Duct of Wirsung:

- Not always seen
- When seen, measure it and put color flow on

Pictured as the line above

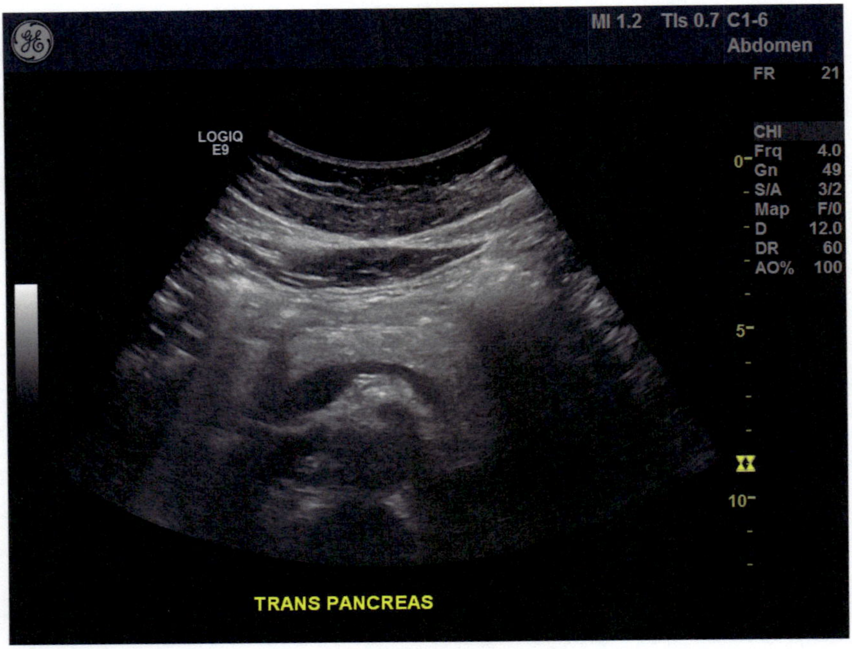

TRV pancreas

<u>Spleen:</u>

When measuring the spleen, keep in mind that some are long and skinny, measuring >12cm. But they are actually normal! This is why taking a splenic volume really helps in determining if the spleen is considered WNL (within normal limits) or if we should classify it as splenomegaly (an enlarged spleen).

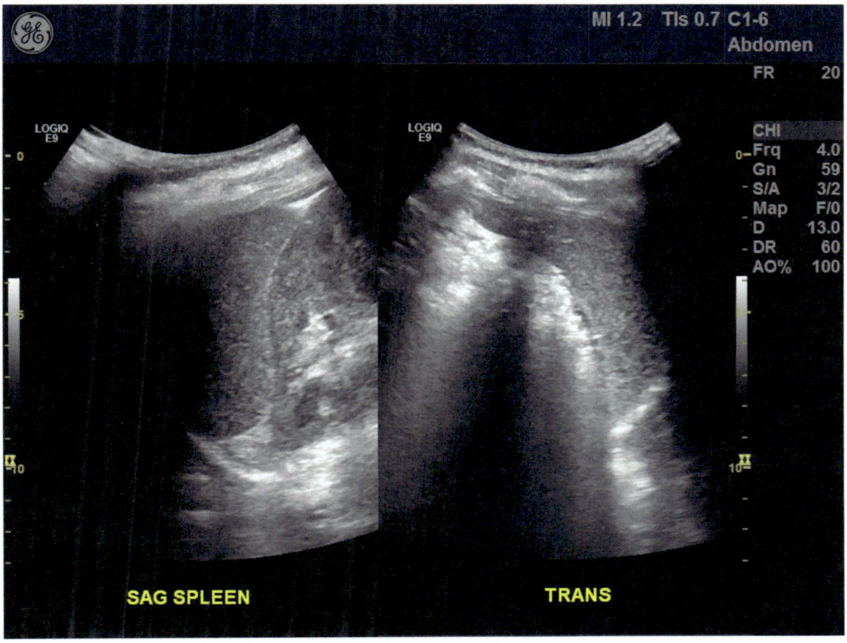

SAG + TRV spleen

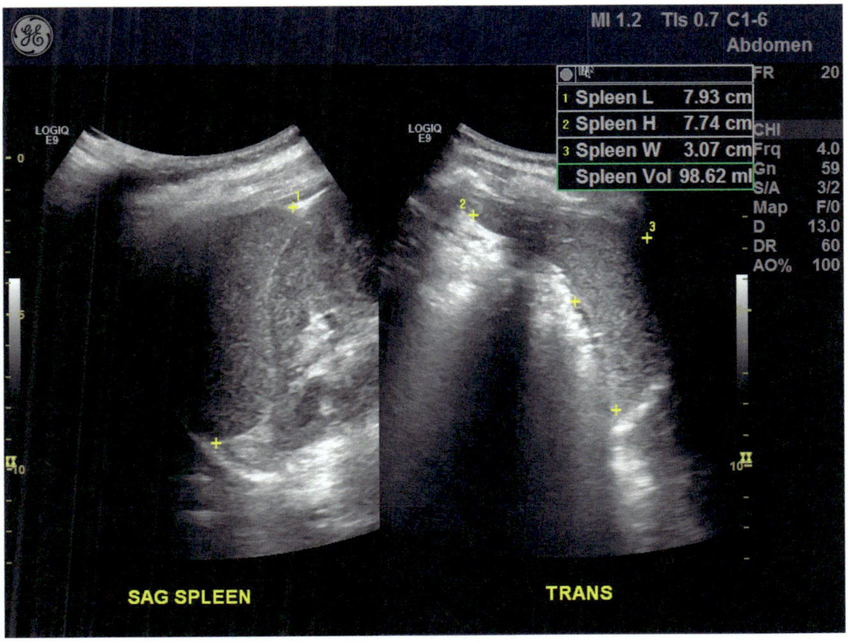

SAG + TRV spleen with measurements

Normal Measurments

Structure:	Abbreviation/ Acronym:	Measurement:
Aorta	AO	<3cm
Appendix	Appy	AP: <6mm
Bladder Wall	BL Wall	**Pre-void / Distended:** <3mm **Post-void / Non-distended:** <5mm (Not an "accurate" measurement for wall thickening)
Common Bile Duct	CBD	<7mm 1mm/decade of age Decade of age + 1mm starting at age 60 Ex: Pt is 60yrs old = 6 - 7mm Ex: Pt is 70yrs old = 7 - 8mm Post Cholecystectomy: normally up to 1cm
Common Pancreatic Duct **Duct of Wirsung**		Head: <3mm Body: <2mm
Gallbladder	GB	**Non-contracted:** L: 7-10cm W: 3-4cm Wall: <3mm
Kidneys	RK + LK	L: 9-13cm AP: 3-6cm W: 4-6cm

Normal Measurements Continued

Structure:	Abbreviation/ Acronym:	Measurement:
Liver	LIV	12-16cm
Pancreas	PANC	**AP:** Head: 2-3cm Neck: 1.5-2.5cm Body: 2-3cm Tail: 1-2cm **Length:** 12-18cm
Spleen	SPL	L: <14cm Vol: <500ml *Many locations use L: <12cm. *Some spleens may be long and thin, measuring >12cm, and that is normal

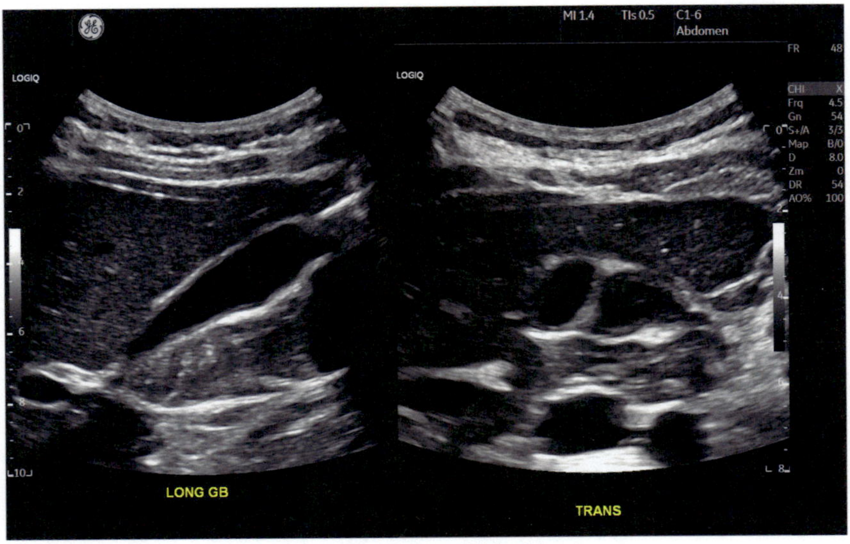

SAG + TRV gallbladder

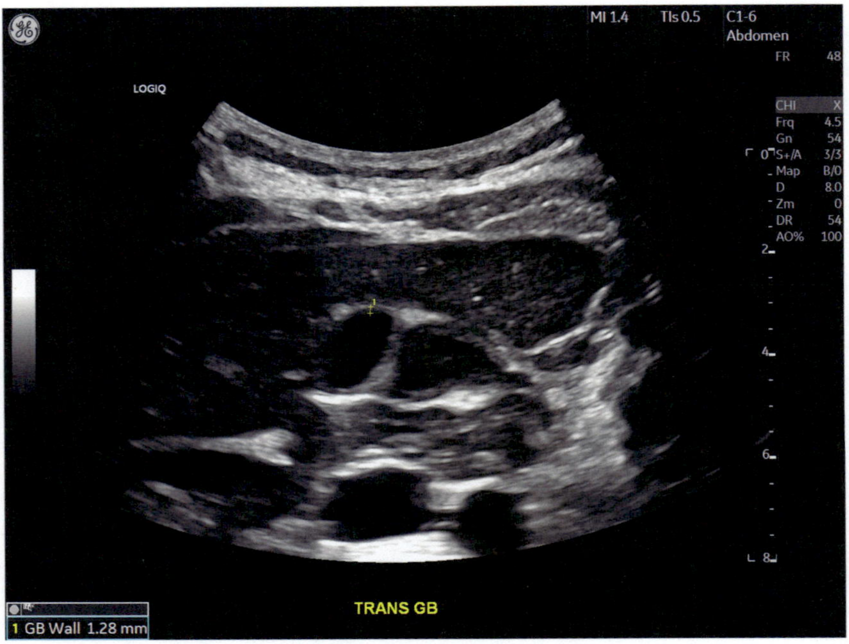

TRV gallbladder wall measurement

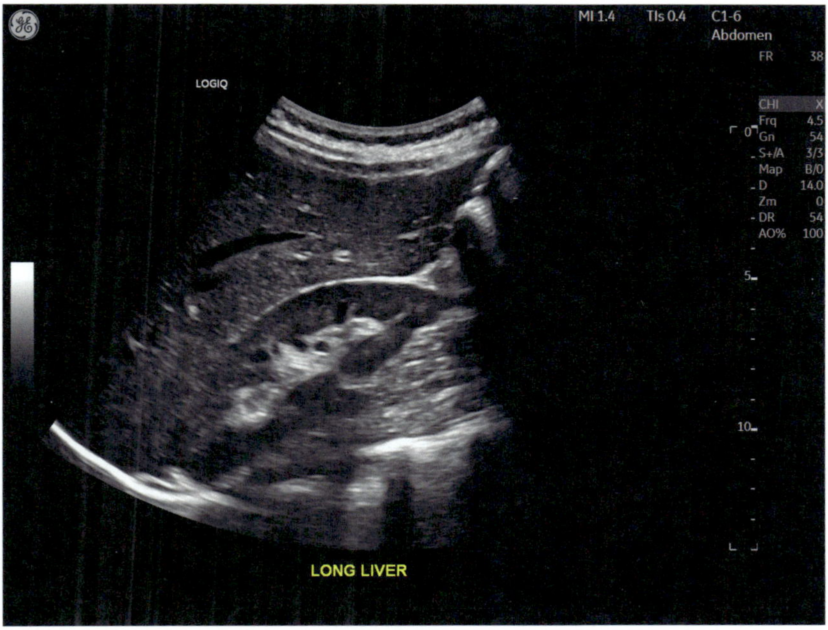

SAG liver

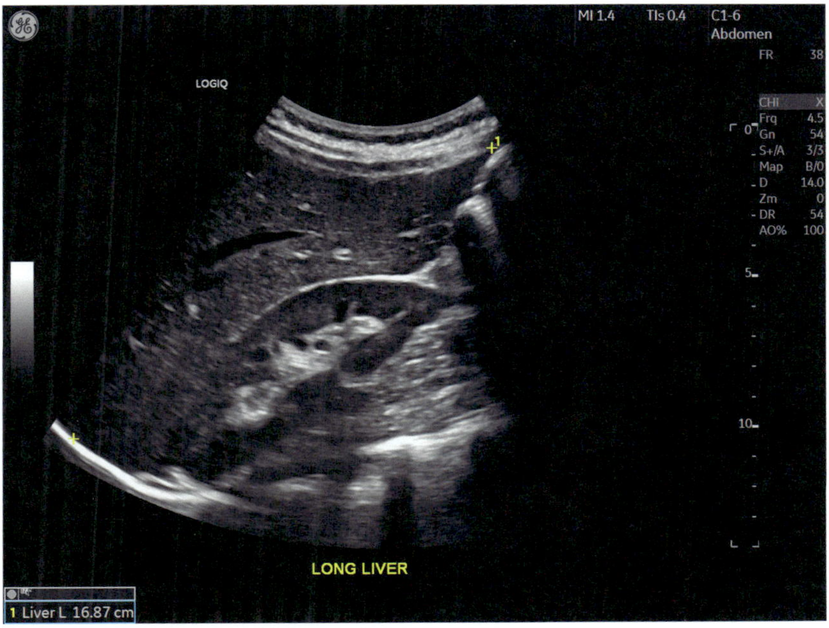

SAG liver with measurement

Protocols

Abdomen Complete:

1. SAG/TRV AO: P + M + D
   a. 2D
   b. Measurements: AP + W
2. SAG IVC
   a. 2D
   b. Color Doppler
   c. Spectral Doppler
3. TRV/SAG Pancreas
4. SAG Liver
   a. 2D: Subcostal/Intercostal
   b. Measurements: L (with the RK in the image)
5. TRV Liver
   a. 2D: Subcostal/Intercostal
6. MPV
   a. Color Doppler
   b. Spectral Doppler
7. HVs
   a. Color Doppler
8. SAG/TRV GB
   a. 2D: Supine + LLD
   b. Measurements: AP wall measurement in TRV
9. CBD
   a. Measurements: AP (with color Doppler on. The CBD will not fill with color)
10. SAG RK
    a. 2D: ML
    b. Measurements: L
    c. Color Doppler
    d. 2D: M-L
11. TRV RK
    a. 2D: Sup
    b. Mid
       i. 2D
       ii. Measurements: AP + W
       iii. Color Doppler
    c. 2D: Inf
12. SAG Liver/Spleen (dual-screen)
13. SAG Spleen
    a. 2D
    b. Measurements: L
14. TRV Spleen
    a. 2D
    b. Measurements: AP + W (calculate a volume)
15. LK (same protocol as the RK)

Document any pathology after getting your protocol images of the organ first

I bet you noticed that in this protocol, after imaging the RK, that you then move on to the spleen instead of the LK. I like to do it this way because it allows separation between the two kidneys. I want to eliminate all possibilities of confusing the radiologist about which kidney they are looking at. Rads are very smart individuals, but they have a lot of cases to read. Therefore, I want to make it easier on them any way I can, and I feel like this can help!

Protocols

Abdomen Limited:

This is the same protocol as the abdomen complete, minus the spleen and LK

Aorta

Patient Prep and Exam

The patient needs to be NPO for 8 hours prior to their exam. Eating and drinking causes bowel gas, obscuring the image quality of the organs and vessels.

Transducers Used

Curvilinear C1-6

Exam Indications

- Hx of tobacco use
- Pulsating mass
- Thoracic aortic aneurysm
- Atheroemboli in the lower extremities
- Known AAA

Normal Measurements

AAA Exam:	Abbreviation / Acronym:	Measurements:	Velocities:	Resistance:
Aorta	AO	<3.0cm	100-150cm/s	Prox + Mid: Low Dist: High
Common Iliac Artery	CIA	<1.5cm	<150cm/s	High
Inferior Vena Cava	IVC	2.5-3.2cm	10-45cm/s	Pulsatile (near the heart)

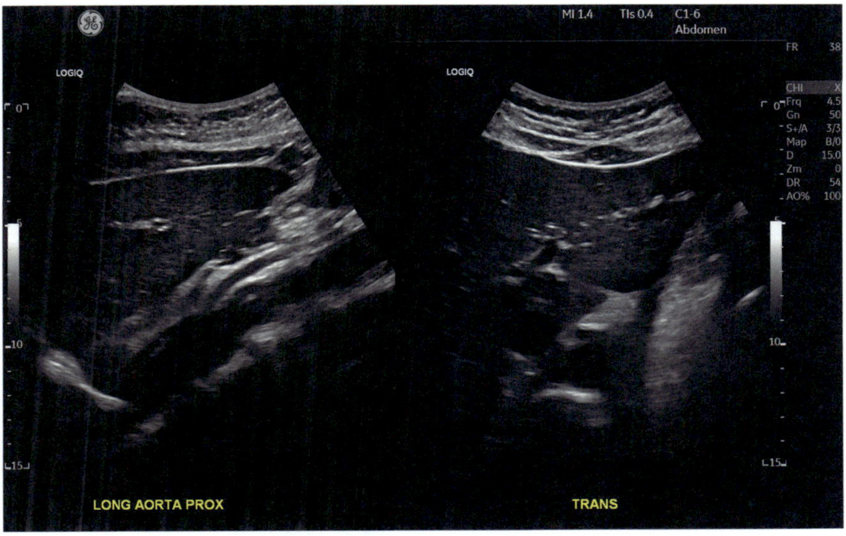

SAG + TRV proximal aorta

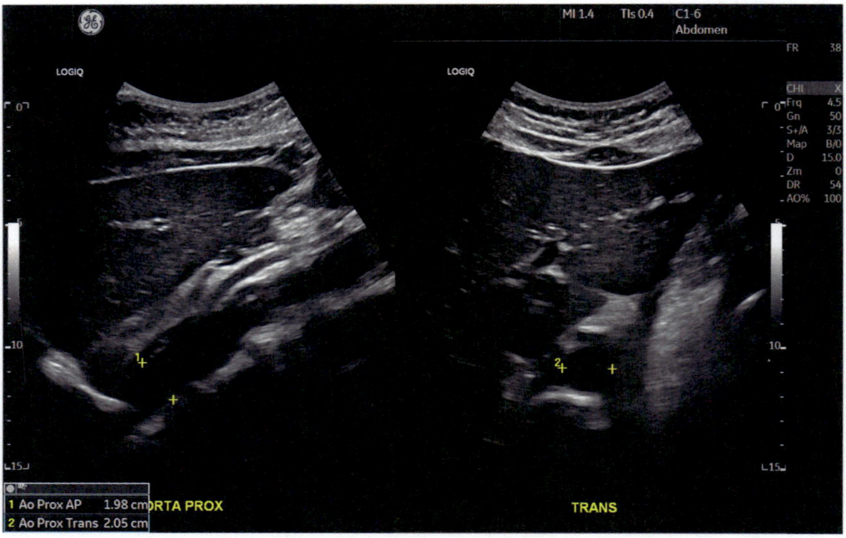

SAG + TRV proximal aorta with measurements

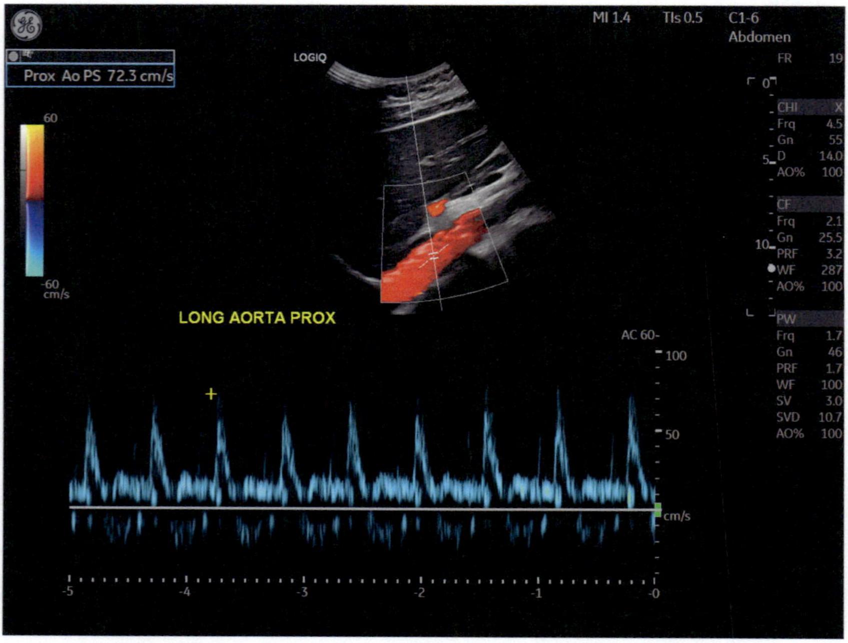

SAG proximal aorta evaluated with color and spectral Doppler

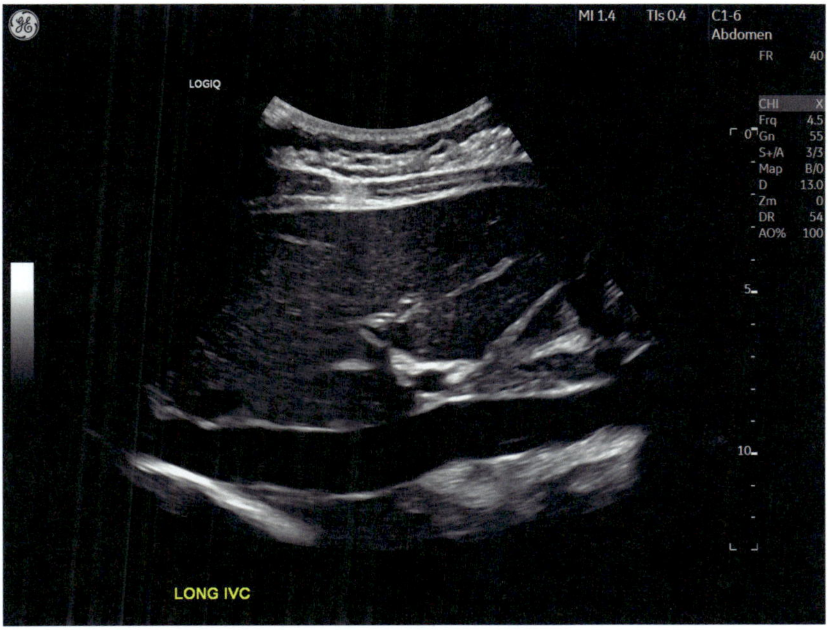

SAG IVC

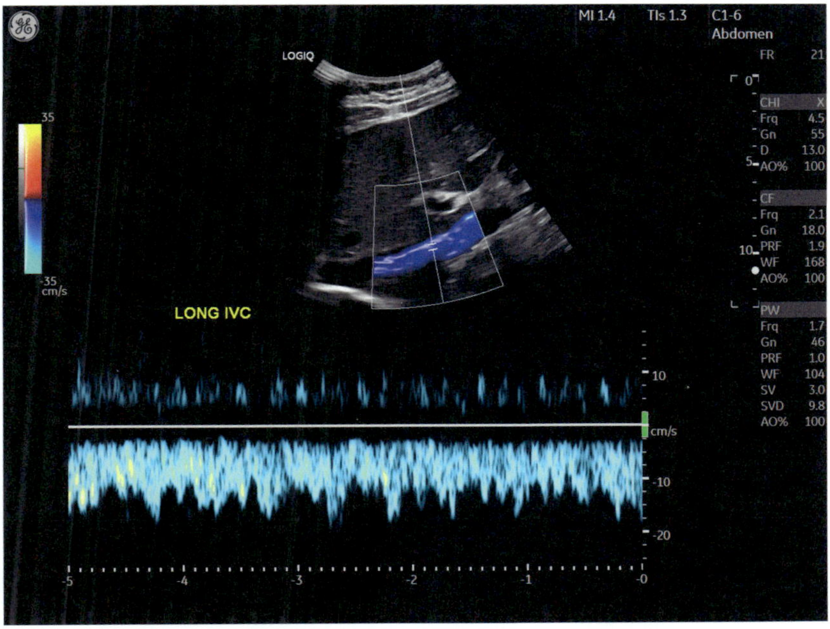

SAG IVC evaluated with color and spectral Doppler

Protocols

Aorta:

1. SAG AO P
   a. 2D
   b. Measurements: AP
2. TRV AO P
   a. 2D
   b. Measurements: W
3. SAG AO M
   a. 2D
   b. Measurements: AP
4. TRV AO M
   a. 2D
   b. Measurements: W
5. SAG AO D
   a. 2D
   b. Measurements: AP
6. TRV AO D
   a. 2D
   b. Measurements: W
7. TRV AO BIF

Make sure to document any pathology along the way. If you see an aneurysm, document the L, AP, and W of it. Include color and spectral Doppler as well

Dual-screen images

7. SAG RT CIA/TRV
   a. 2D
   b. Measurements: AP on SAG image, W on TRV image
8. SAG LT CIA/TRV
   a. 2D
   b. Measurements: AP on SAG image, W on TRV image

Document with color and spectral Doppler

9. SAG IVC
10. SAG AO P
11. SAG AO M
12. SAG AO D
13. SAG RT CIA
14. SAG LT CIA

Renal

Patient Prep and Examination

The patient needs to arrive with full bladder. We evaluate the bladder as part of the protocol. If the bladder is not distended, we won't be able to determine if there is pathology or not.

Transducers Used

- Renal: Curvilinear C1-6
- Prostate: C1-6

Exam Indications

- Flank px
- Hematuria
- Dysuria
- Recurrent UTIs
- CKD
- AKI

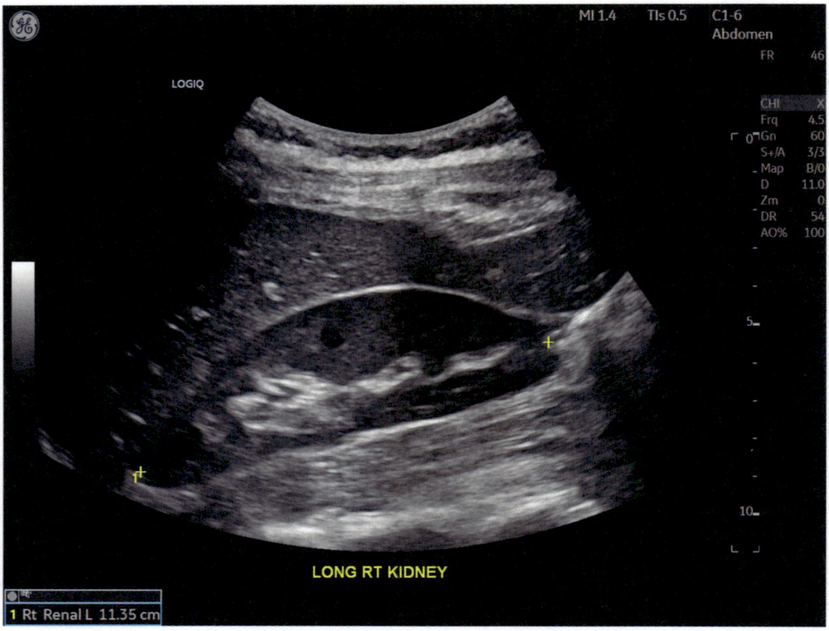

SAG right kidney with measurements

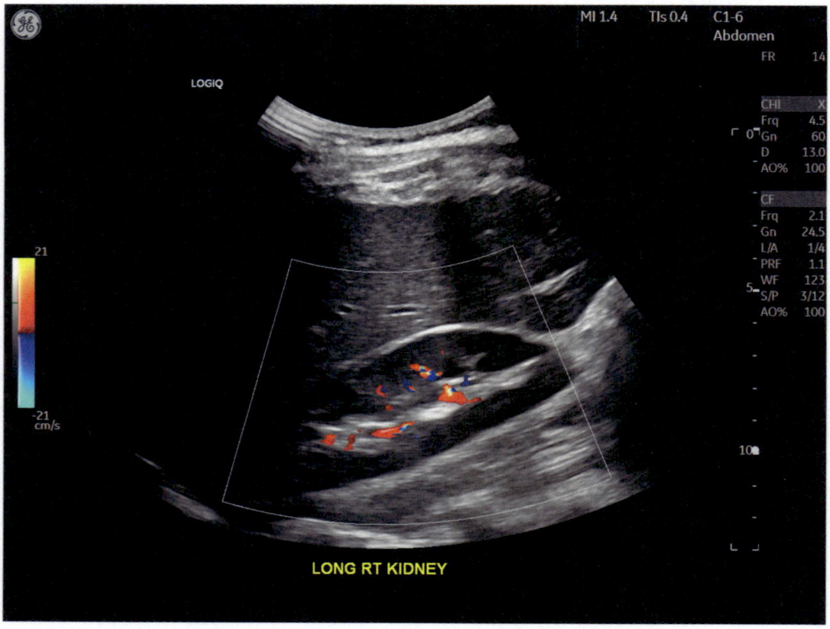

SAG right kidney evaluated with color Doppler

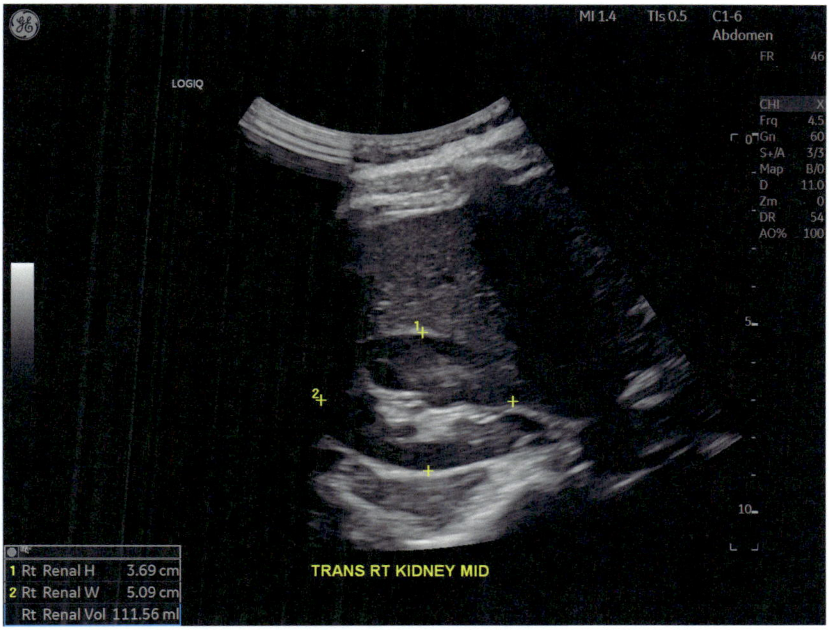

TRV mid right kidney

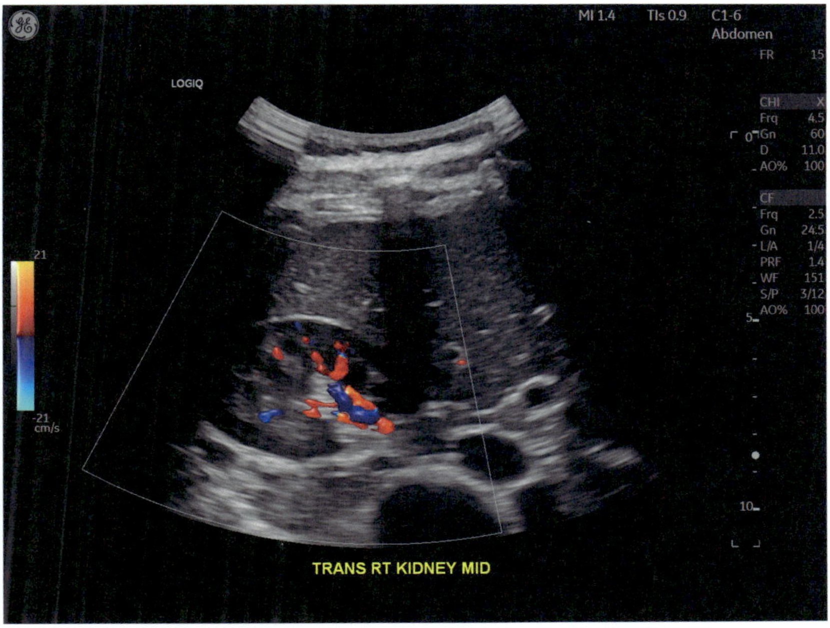

TRV mid right kidney evaluated with color Doppler

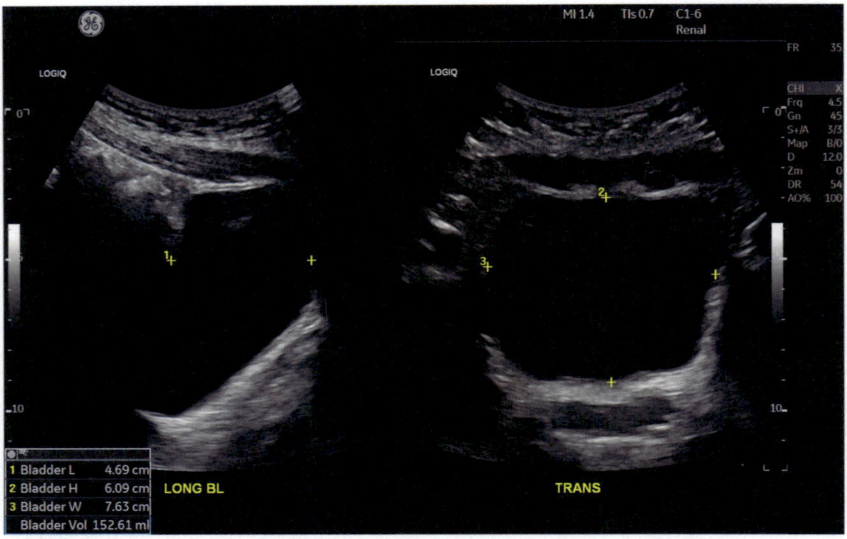

SAG + TRV bladder with measurements

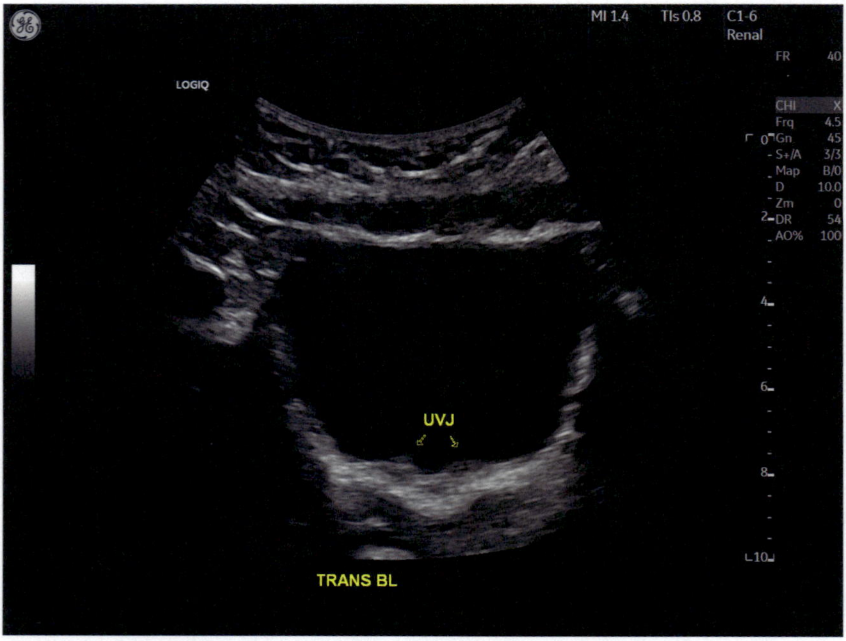

TRV bladder showing the ureterovesical junctions

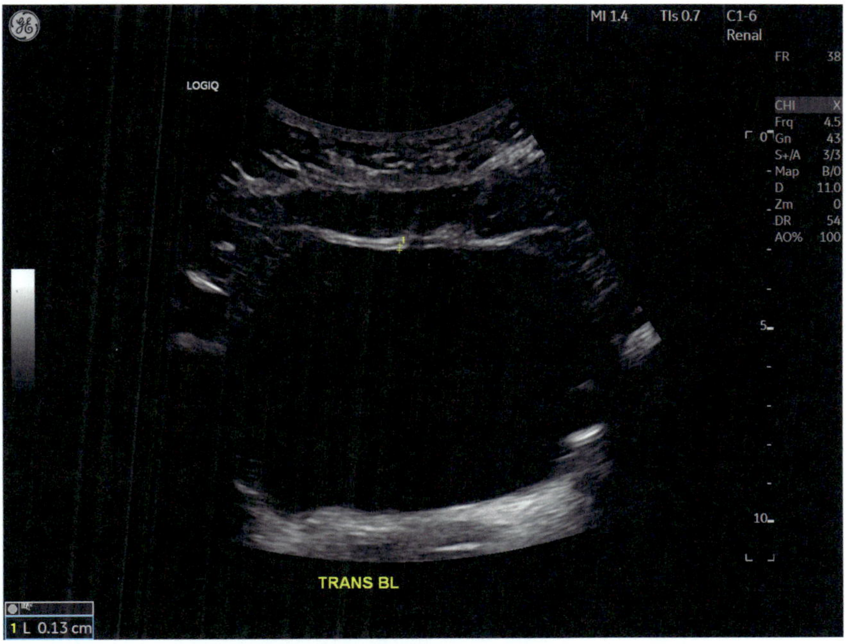

TRV bladder wall measurement

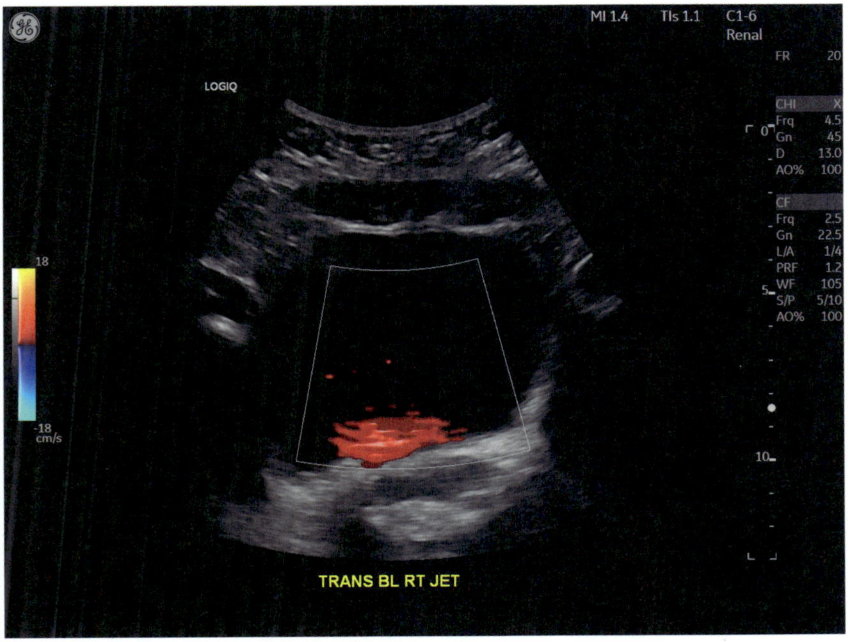

Bladder jet: right

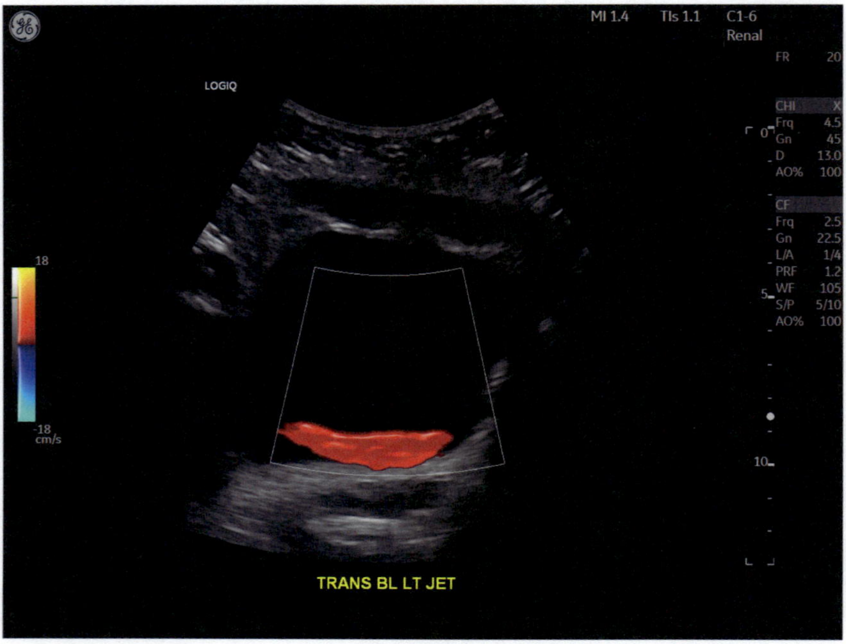

Bladder jet: Left

Protocols

Renal:

1. SAG RK
    a. 2D: ML
    b. Measurements: L
    c. Color Doppler
    d. 2D: M-L
2. TRV RK
    a. 2D: Sup
    b. Mid
        i. 2D
        ii. Measurements: AP + W
        iii. Color Doppler
    c. 2D: Inf
3. LK (same protocol as the RK)
4. SAG/TRV BL
    a. 2D
    b. Measurements: L + AP + W (calculate a volume)
5. TRV BL
    a. Document both bladder jets
6. SAG/TRV PROST (dual-image)
    a. 2D
    b. Measurements: L + AP + W (calculate a volume)
    c. Color Doppler

If the patient is male, include the prostate in the protocol

If the patient is male, include the prostate in this exam. Document the prostate when the patient has a full bladder. It is quite difficult to visualize the prostate if the bladder is not distended. I have caught prostate cancer a time or two by doing this.

Notes

Notes

Notes

2

Breast

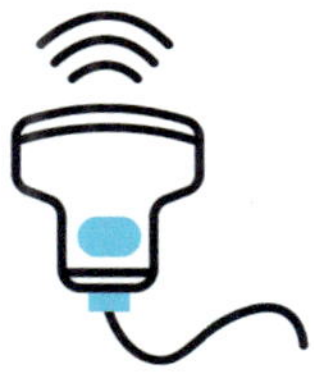

Patient Prep and Exam

There is no patient prep prior to this exam. At the appointment, the only thing the patient needs to do is take their shirt and bra off and change into a gown.

Transducers Used

- ML6-15
- On occasion, I have used the curvilinear C1-6 on large breast implants

Exam Indications

- Yearly screening
- Asymmetry seen on mammo

- Px
- Lump
- High risk or hx of BR CA
- Nipple discharge
- Skin discoloration and/or itching

Functions

Structure:	Function:
Glandular Tissue	Dense tissue made up of lobules that produce milk
Lactiferous Ducts	Carries milk from the lobules to the nipple
Nipple	The lactiferous ducts accumulate here, allowing milk to pass through for breastfeeding

Normal Measurements

Structure:	Measurement:
Lactiferous Ducts	Not Pregnant: <3mm Pregnant/Nursing: <8mm
Skin	2mm

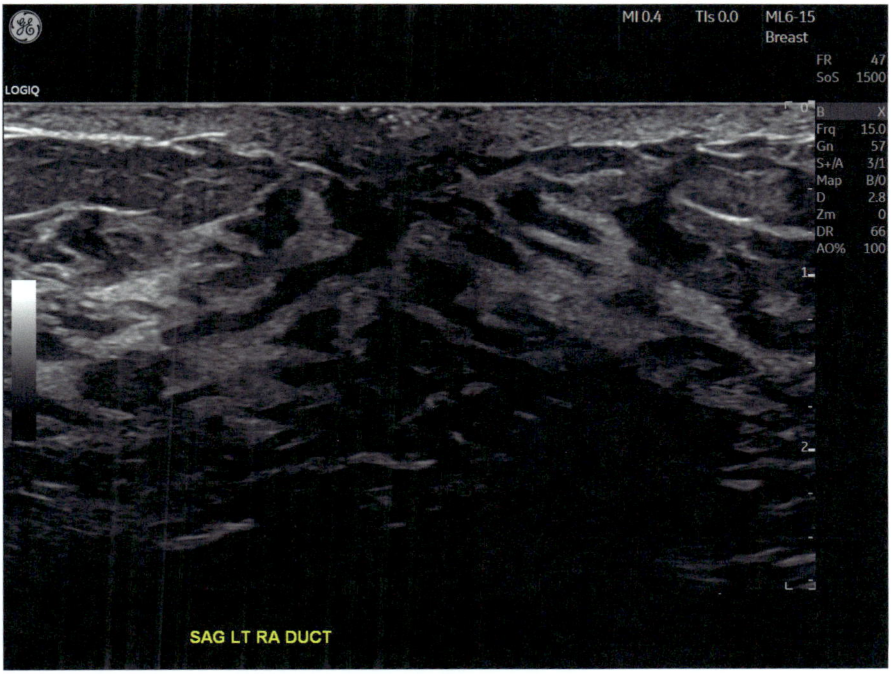

A duct posterior the the left nipple

Screening Mammograms

Patients will start screening mammos (mammograms) at age 40. This can be subject to change, as we have decreased the screening age over the years. We have done this because we are finding that more women are having breast cancer at earlier ages.

Patients can start their screening mammos earlier if they have had BR (breast) CA (cancer) before or if they are at a higher risk. For example, the patient would be at higher risk if their mother, grandmother, or sister had BR CA at age 32.

Breasts are made up of many different tissue layers. One of those layers is glandular tissue or mammary glands. This tissue is responsible for producing milk. Glandular tissue on mammo shows up as "white" and can obscure masses. This is because masses also present as "white". However, on US (ultrasound), we can see through that dense tissue and visualize/characterize masses.

Tissue Layers - In Descending Order

Female:	Male:
• Skin • Subcutaneous fat • Glandular Tissue • Retroglandular fat • Pectoralis muscles • Ribs + Intercostal muscle • Pleura • Lung	• Skin • Subcutaneous fat • Pectoralis muscles • Ribs + Intercostal muscle • Pleura • Lung

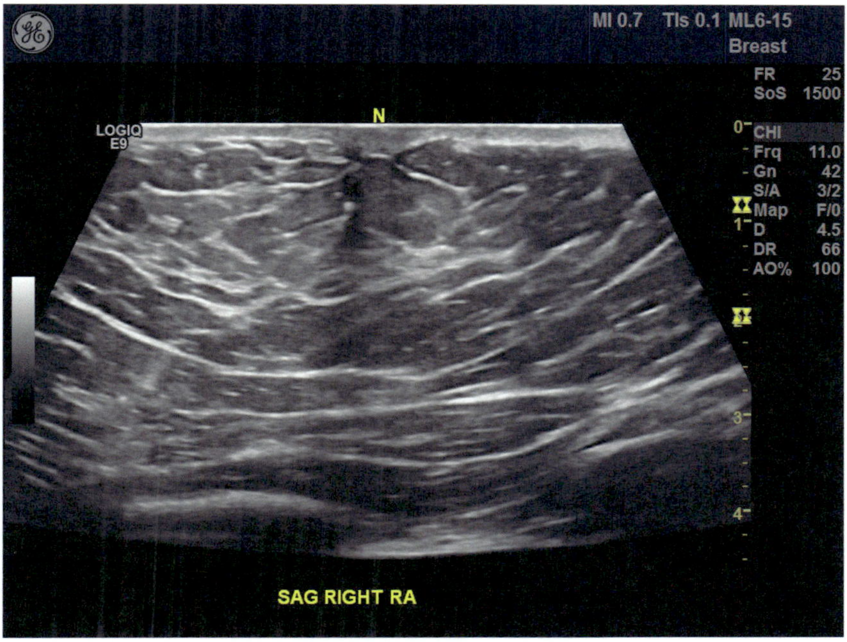

Male breast. N: Nipple

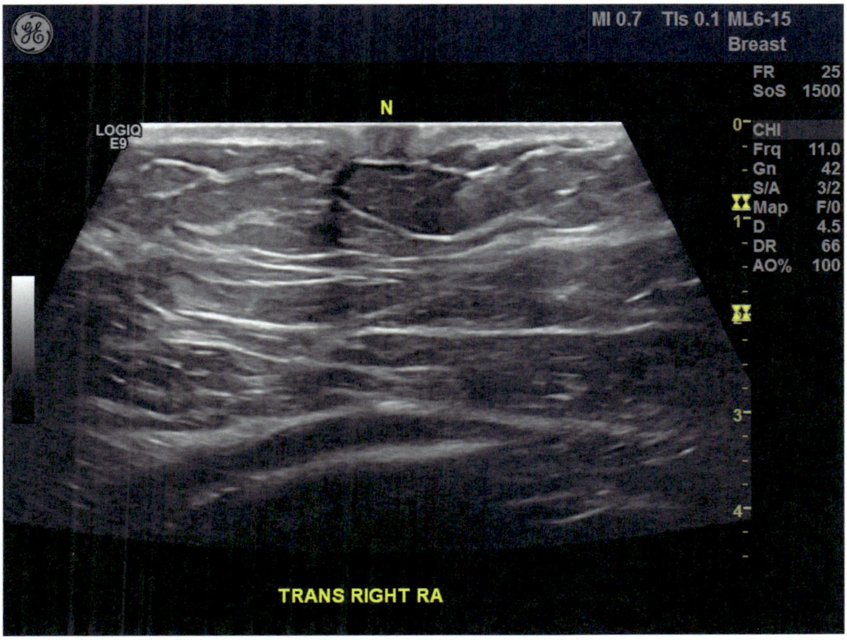

Male breast. N: Nipple

One of the main reasons why we start mammo screenings at age 40 is because this is when glandular tissue starts to become replaced by fat. Fat on mammo shows up as "gray" making it easier to so see any and all "white" masses. Before age 30, women's breast tissue is considerably dense, making mammos more challenging to diagnose any pathology.

Breast Density Levels

Level:	%:	Meaning:	Notes:
1	<25%	Predominantly fat	No glandular tissue
2	25-50%	Scattered fibroglandular tissue	Some glandular tissue / islands of glandular tissue
3	50-75%	Heterogeneously dense	Moderate amount of glandular tissue
4	>75%	Extremely dense	Mostly glandular tissue

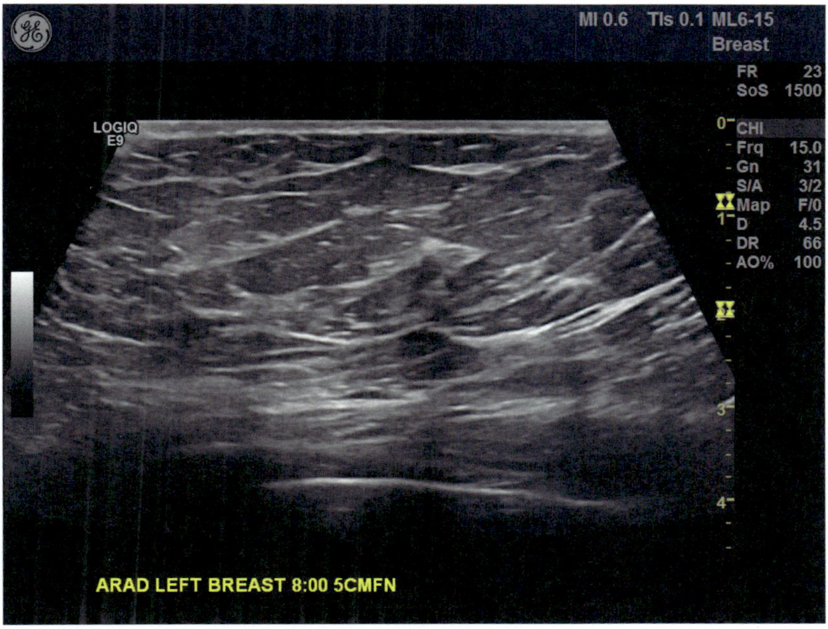

Breast density level 1

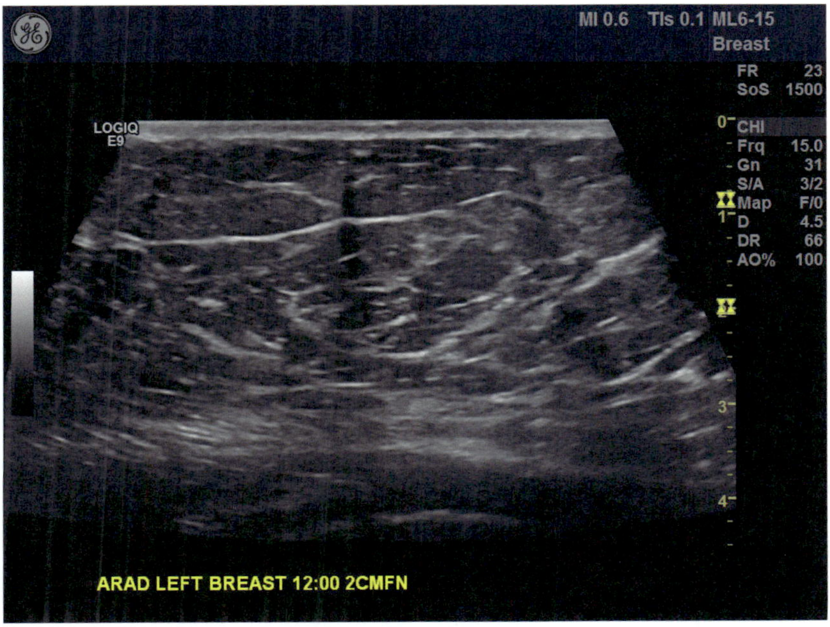

Breast density level 1

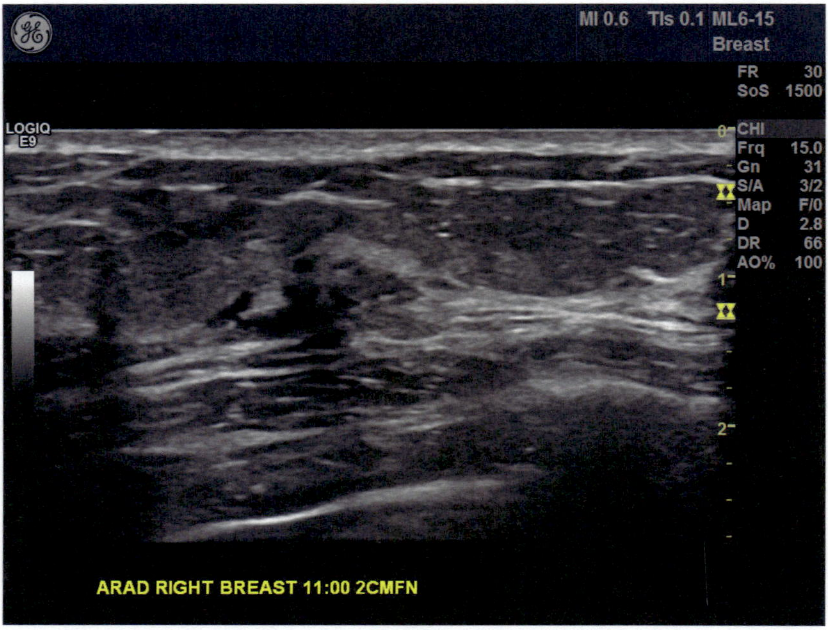

Breast density level 2: Island of glandular tissue

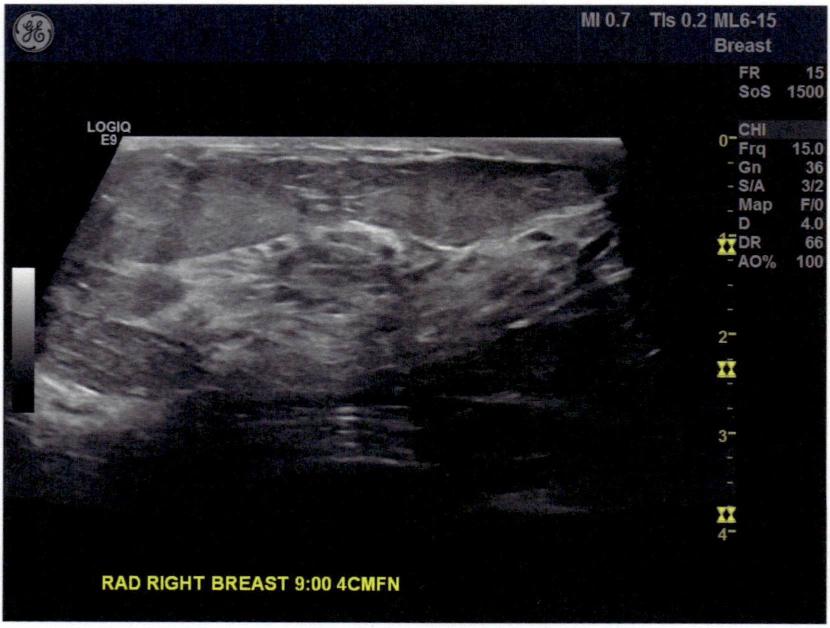

Breast density level 3

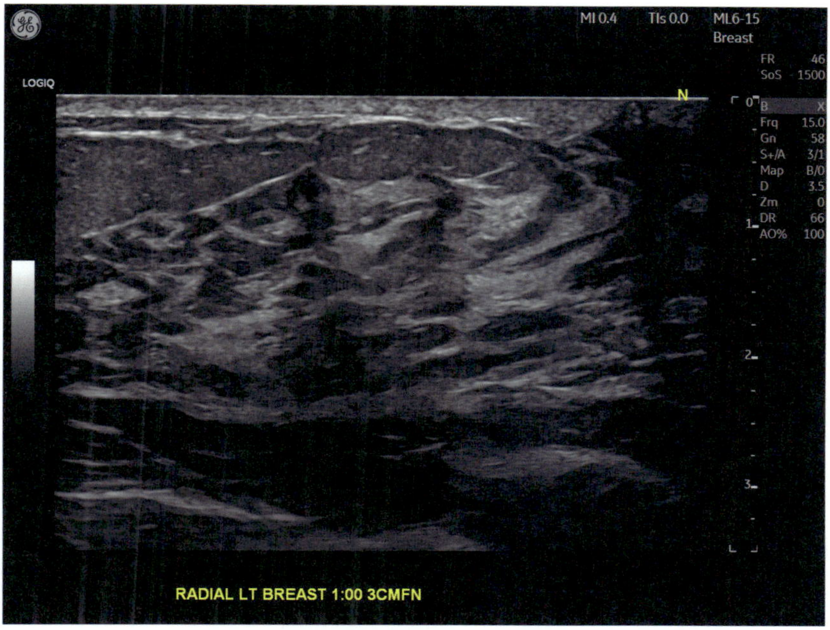

Breast density level 4

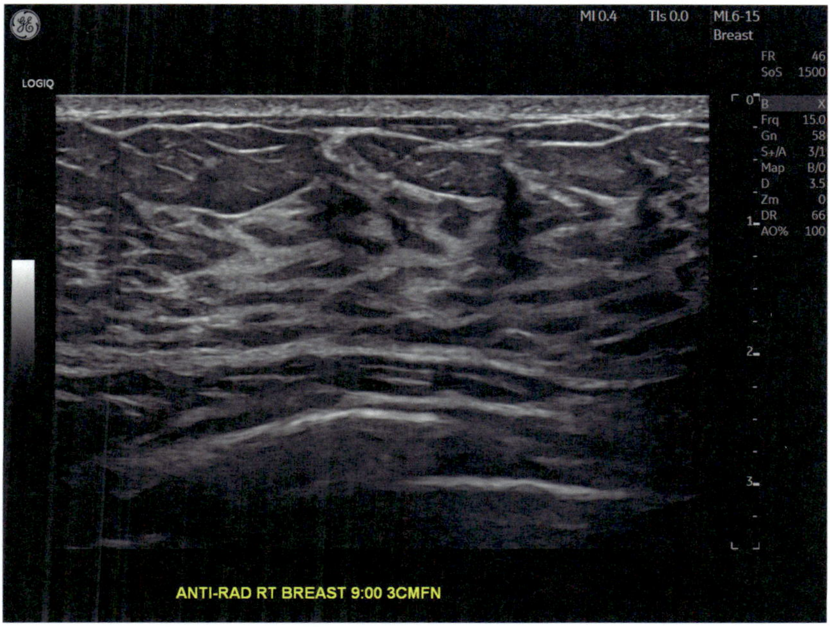

Breast density level 4

Mammo, US, or Both?

So how do we decide if a patient needs a mammo, US, or both? Well, let's take a look. Let's say that we have 2 patients; one patient is UNDER the age of 30 and one is OVER the age of 30. Both patients have a breast lump. Automatically, this is considered a diagnostic ultrasound and a diagnostic mammogram because the lump is palpable and the patient will have both ordered. However, just because they are both ordered, does not necessarily mean that the patient will have both exams done. Here's why...

- Patient UNDER 30: Scheduled in US first, then mammo second (due to the patient most likely having dense breast tissue)
  - If the US is negative, meaning the breast is normal and no "lump" or pathology is seen, then the mammo can be canceled. If we do find pathology, then the mammo will be done
- Patient OVER 30: Scheduled as a mammo first, then US second
  - If the mammo is negative; again, meaning nothing was found, the patient will still get an US. This is because of breast imaging guidelines. We want to confirm with US that no "lump" or pathology is seen
  - If the "lump" is seen on mammo, as in we see pathology corresponding to the patient's symptom, then the patient will have the ultrasound to characterize the mass

Now let's say that these two patients don't have lumps, but they have px (pain) instead. Again, this is considered a diagnostic US and a diagnostic mammo.

- Patient UNDER 30: Scheduled as US first, then mammo second (due to the patient most likely having dense breast tissue)
    - If the US is negative, then the mammo is not needed. But if we find pathology, then the patient will have the mammo
- Patient OVER 30: Scheduled as a mammo first, then US second
    - If the mammo is negative, but the patient has focal (localized area) pain, then the US will be done
    - If the mammo is negative, but the patient has global (the entire breast or a large area) pain, then the US can be canceled
    - If the mammo is positive, meaning we find pathology, then the US will be performed to characterize the mass

Global pain is a more benign symptom, where focal is considered more concerning. This is why focal pain will be evaluated with ultrasound and global pain will be canceled.

When patients come in with pain or lumps, we are only imaging the AOC (area of concern). We don't typically perform screening ultrasounds on patients with these types of symptoms.

Screening US + MRIs

Going back to breast density, keep in mind that NOT ALL women lose their glandular tissue at age 40. Some women will still have VERY dense breasts even in their 90s! Dense breasts in women in their 90s is rare, but it still can happen. Because of this, some women will need a screening US in ADDITION to their screening mammo. Screening ultrasounds are also performed on women who have had breast cancer before.

Sometimes screening mammos and screening ultrasounds can be performed on the same day, but some providers like to space them out. For example, the screening mammo will be done, then 6 months later the screening ultrasound will be done. 6 months after the ultrasound, the patient will have another screening mammo. Doing it this way, the patient is still only getting one mammo and one ultrasound per year, but is getting imaged in 6 month intervals. This allows for closer evaluation of high risk patients.

Some women will have screening MRIs in addition to their screening mammos and ultrasounds. However, in order to get a screening MRI, a patient has to be considered high risk, have very dense breast tissue, or have had breast cancer before.

Mammo, US, or Both?

Screening

PT Age:	Notes:	Imaging Needed:
40+	No symptoms	Mammo
40+	Very dense High risk	Mammo + US
<40	High risk Hx of BR CA Mother had BR CA diagnosed under 40	Mammo + US Possibly screening MRI

Lump

PT Age:	1st Exam:	Path Found:	2nd Exam Needed:
<30	US	No	Cx
<30	US	Yes	Mammo
>30	Mammo	No	US
>30	Mammo	Yes	US

Mammo, US, or Both?

Pain <30

PT Age:	1st Exam:	Px Location:	Path Found:	Mammo Needed?
<30	US	Focal	No	✗
<30	US	Focal	Yes	✓
<30	US	Global	No	✗
<30	US	Global	Yes	✓

Pain >30

PT Age:	1st Exam:	Px Location:	Path Found:	US Needed?
>30	Mammo	Focal	No	✓
>30	Mammo	Focal	Yes	✓
>30	Mammo	Global	No	✗
>30	Mammo	Global	Yes	✓

Radiation!?

Let's briefly discuss radiation, as this is a very common topic of conversation within the breast imaging world.

- US DOES NOT use radiation. We use sonographic waves.
- MRI DOES NOT use radiation, but a giant magnet instead.
- Mammo DOES use radiation, however, it is a very low dose. In fact, you are consistently exposed to more radiation in your everyday life than a mammo will ever give you. In fact, the 3D mammo machines produce less radiation than the older 2D machines.

Some people are very concerned about the amount of radiation that a mammo machine emits. But as I said above, it's actually not that much. This misunderstanding can cause people to decline screening mammos and have a screening US instead. This is not recommended. Mammos are excellent at finding pre-cancer in the form of microcalcifications. Ultrasound, unfortunately, can't see those microcalcifications. Cancer has to be a little further along, in the form of a mass for US to see it. Another note to add is that there are some cancers that only mammo can pick up. Therefore, mammo is the gold standard for breast cancer screening and US is fantastic for mass characterization.

Setting Up the Image

We use "radial" and "antiradial" in breast imaging as well as sagittal and transverse. In short form, they are called RAD and ARAD or ANTI-RAD. Rad is more like SAG and ARAD is more like TRV, however, they are not exactly the same! Think of radial like rays of the sun. The position of the transducer is that the head or toe (short side) of the transducer points towards the nipple. Antiradial, on the other hand, is exactly perpendicular to radial. The long, flat side of the transducer faces towards the nipple.

Given this description, while imaging in the radial plane, the transducer notch DOESN'T ALWAYS face towards the nipple. Let me explain.

- 1:00-6:00 – Notch is pointed TOWARDS the nipple
- 7:00-12:00 – Notch is pointed AWAY from the nipple

One of the reasons why we do this is because of ergonomics. You would be straining your wrist and twisting your body if you always had the notch pointed towards the nipple. If you don't turn your body into a pretzel, you would have to completely turn the transducer around in your hand, which is not ergonomical, correct, or efficient. Another reason we do this is because if we always had the notch pointed towards the nipple, the mass would appear to be backward half the time.

RAD + ARAD

RT BR

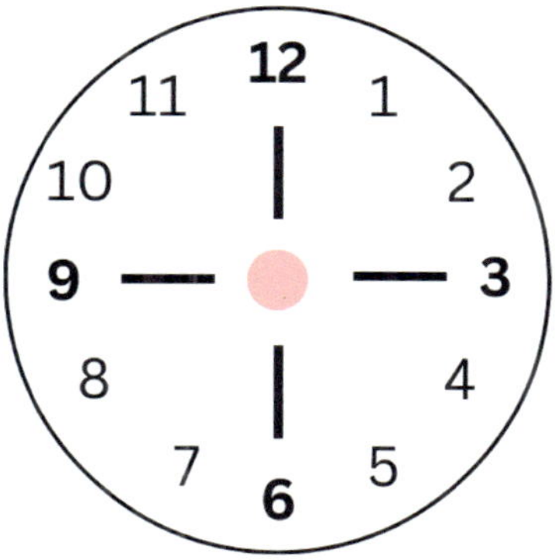

LT BR

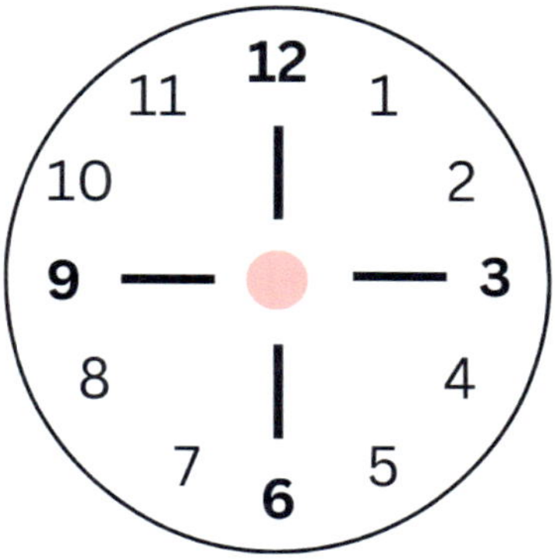

We think of the breast as a clock. The clock is the same set-up on both breasts!

RAD

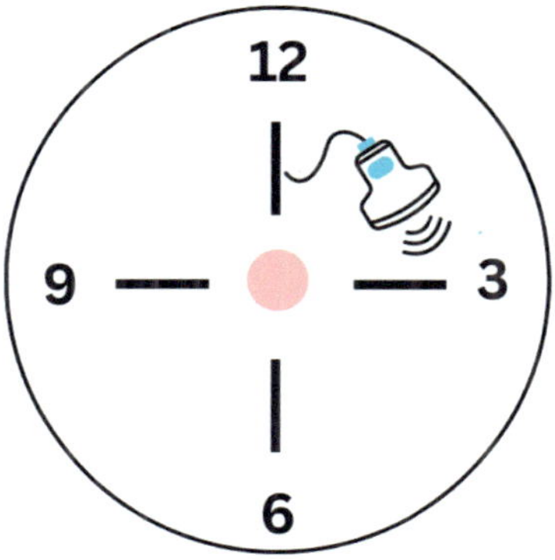

Radial: The head or toe of the transducer should be pointing towards the nipple

ARAD

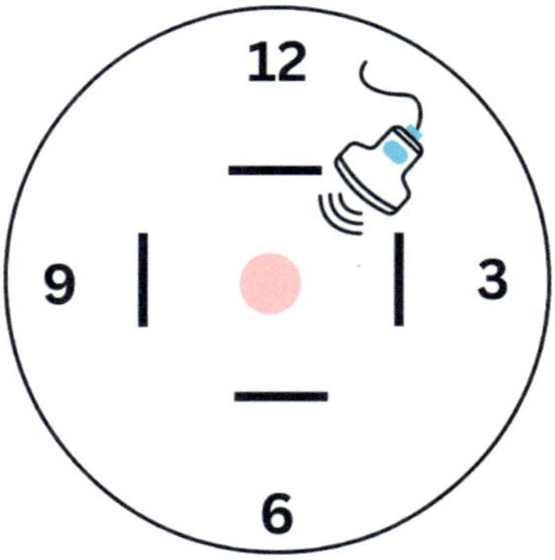

Antiradial: The long, flat side should be facing towards the nipple

Annotations

Breast

How do we annotate images that are related to the breast (not axilla or retroareolar)? We annotate in this order:

- RAD or ARAD
- RIGHT or LEFT
- BREAST
- O'clock position
- CMFN

EX 1: Let's say that we have a mass in the right breast at 2:00, 3CMFN but we want to image it in radial. We would annotate as such: RAD RIGHT BREAST 2:00 3CMFN

EX 2: Let's say that we have a mass in the left breast at 11:00, 8CMFN but we want to image it in antiradial. We would annotate as such: ARAD LEFT BREAST 11:00 8CMFN

Retroareolar

How do we annotate images that are RA (retroareolar)? For the RA, we use SAG and TRV. We would annotate in this order:

- SAG or TRV
- RIGHT or LEFT
- RA

EX 1: Let's say we want to evaluate a mass located in the left RA in SAG. We would annotate as such: SAG LEFT RA

EX 2: Let's say we want to evaluate a mass located in the RIGHT RA in TRV. We would annotate as such: TRV RIGHT RA

Some sonographers will add an "o'clock" position to be even more specific. This can be super helpful when following another sonographer's work, but it is not necessary.

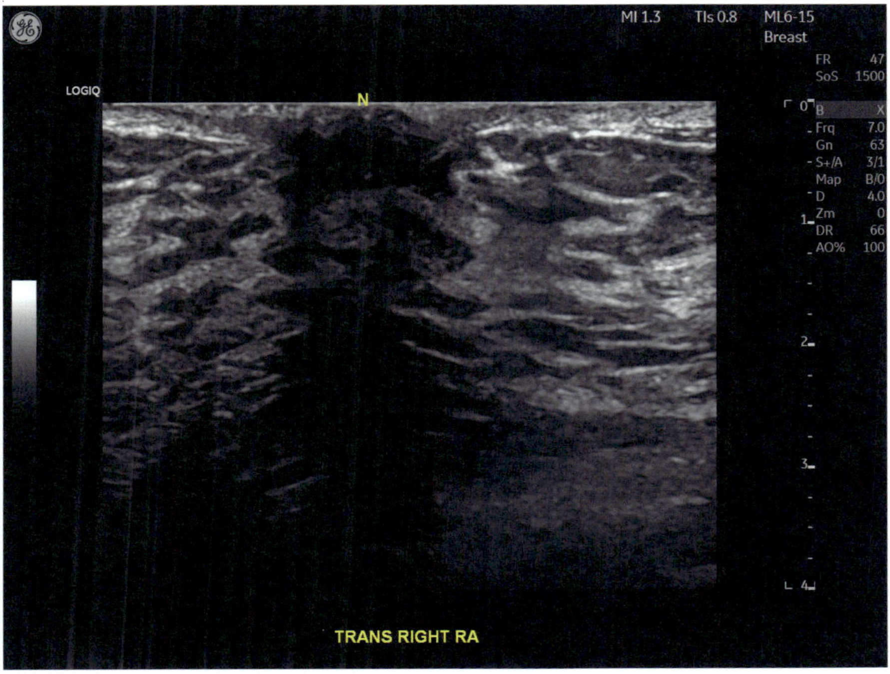

TRV right retroareolar

Axilla

How do we annotate images that are in the axilla? For the axilla, we also use SAG and TRV. We would annotate in this order:

- SAG or TRV
- RIGHT or LEFT
- AXILLA
- SUP, MID, or INF

EX 1: Let's say we want to evaluate a LN (lymph node) in the right superior axilla in SAG. We would annotate as such: SAG RIGHT AXILLA SUP

EX 2: Let's say we want to evaluate a LN in the left inferior axilla in TRV. We would annotate as such: TRV LEFT AXILLA INF

BI-RADS

So how do we determine what masses are benign versus what masses should be biopsied? Well, we grade masses on a BI-RADS scale. We grade them based on echogenicity, vascularity, borders, shape, size, solid vs cystic, etc. Benign masses have different characteristics than cancerous masses.

Once we image the mass, we send our images and worksheet to the rad. The rad then takes a look at our study and gives us a BI-RADS score. If the mass scores a 2 on the BI-RADS scale, then the mass is benign and we don't need to follow it up.

An example of this would be a simple cyst. If the mass scores a 3 on the BI-RADS scale, then we will have the patient return in 6 months for another ultrasound. As a BI-RADS 3, the mass is most likely benign; however, we have the patient return for a follow-up ultrasound to see if the mass changes at all. An example of this kind of mass would be a fibroadenoma.

If the mass scores a 4 or 5, then we believe the mass is malignant and we will be doing an ultrasound-guided biopsy of the mass. The only time a mass gets a score of 6 on the BI-RADS chart is after we biopsy the mass and it comes back from pathology as containing malignant cells. An example of this would be invasive ductal carcinoma.

Scoring a 0 on the BI-RADS chart means that the patient will need further imaging. For instance, if a patient has a lump and only has a mammo scheduled, they will get a BI-RADS 0 and will need to come back for an ultrasound whenever they can get that scheduled. They will get a BI-RADS 0 even if no pathology was identified on the mammo. Because of breast imaging guidelines, the patient will need to come back for the ultrasound.

BI-RADS:

BI-RAD:	Meaning:	% Probability of Malignancy:	Treatment + Follow-up:
0	Incomplete	-	Diagnostic mammo or US
1	Normal Mammo	0%	Yearly screening
2	Benign	0%	Yearly Screening
3	Probably benign	<2%	3 or 6- month short interval follow-up
4	Suspicious for malignancy	4a: Low: 2-10% 4b: Mod: 10-50% 4c: High: 50-95%	Biopsy
5	Highly suspicious for malignancy	>95%	Biopsy
6	Malignant - biopsy proven	100%	Treatment of cancer

Notes

Notes

Notes

3

Liver Elastography

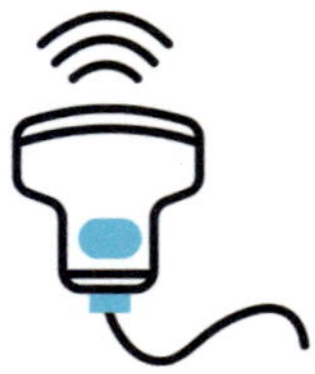

Patient Prep and Exam

The patient needs to be NPO for 8 hours before the exam. Eating and drinking causes bowel gas, obscuring the image quality of the organs and vessels. Not all imaging facilities will do a patient prep for this exam, however, you may be dealing with bowel gas as a consequence.

Transducers Used

- Curvilinear C1-6

Exam Indications

- Hepatic steatosis
- Hep B or Hep C

- ETOH

Sample Box Tips

- Place the box about 1.5-2cm deep to the liver capsule
  - Avoid placing the box and sampling in the posterior liver
  - Avoid sampling greater than 8cm deep – this can become a challenge on larger patients
- Place the box in the right lobe of the liver only. Avoid the left lobe, as samples are less accurate
- Keep the box parallel to the liver capsule
- Place the box only over liver tissue
  - Avoid vessels and ducts (otherwise the color won't fill in – you will have gaps in your sample)
- Use a smaller box for a targeted sample
- Take 12 (or however many your department determines as protocol) samples, each lasting roughly 3 seconds
  - These 12 samples need to be taken consistently in the same spot of the right liver. Don't move the sample box around

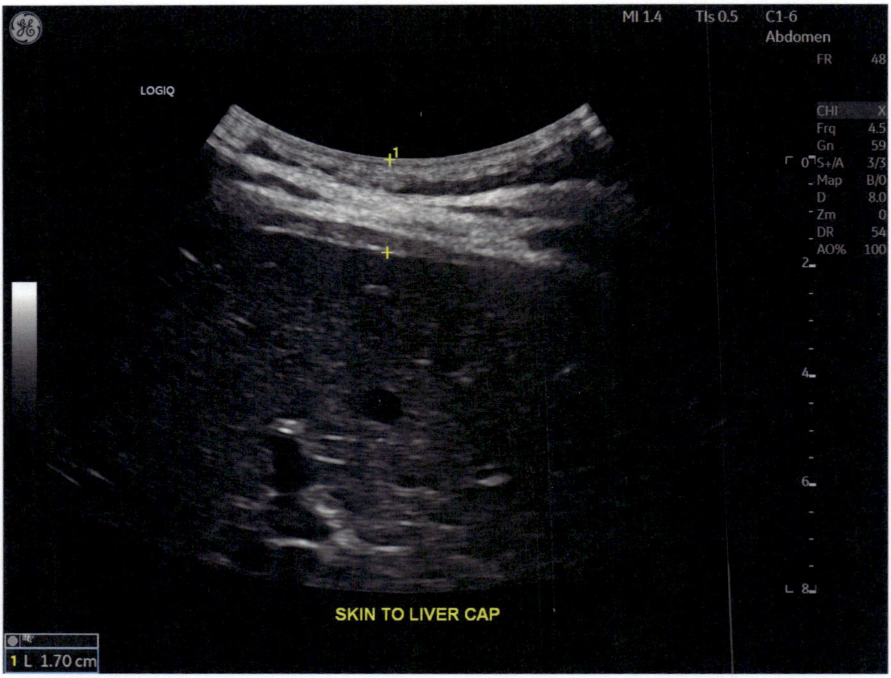

Measurement of the distance between the skin and liver capsule

Sample Box Colors

Color:	Stiffness:	Notes:
Blue	Low	Normal Tissue
Yellow	Moderate	Indicative of liver disease
Red	High	Significant for cirrhosis

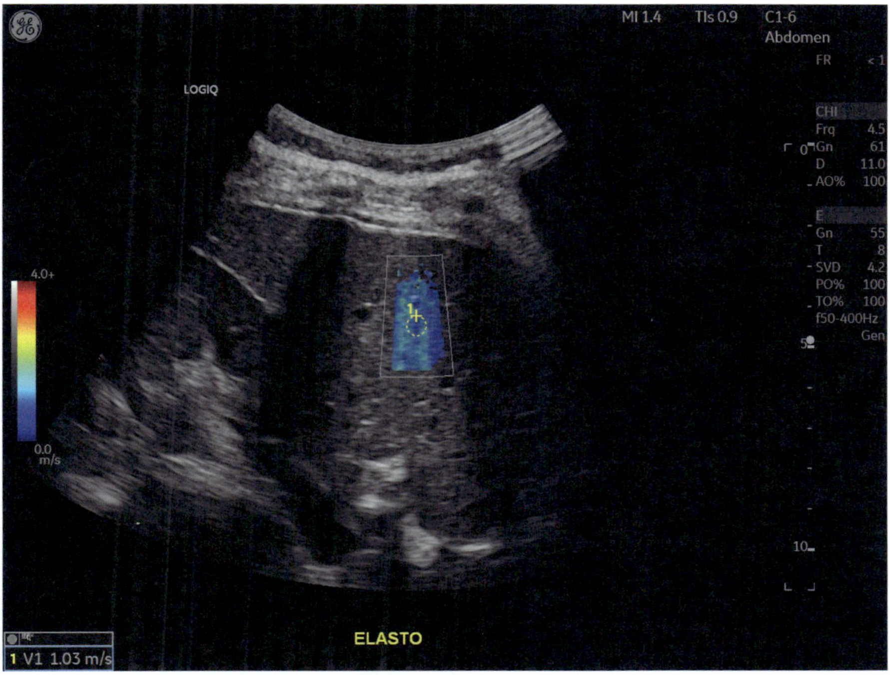

Elastography sample

Helpful Tips

- Patient position: Supine with their right arm relaxed over their head, resting on the pillow
  - If the patient is full of gas, you can LLD the patient but try to keep the patient supine if you can
- Best images are taken in an intercostal approach rather than subcostal. However, the subcostal approach may be utilized, especially for patients with a high BMI or excessive rib shadowing
- Every time a sample is taken, the patient should hold/pause their breathing

  - Breathing motion obscures the sampling and will give you inaccurate results
  - Don't let the patient take a big breath in! It should be a very small breath or they should still their breathing. Large breaths cause intra-abdominal pressure and will obscure the results

Pitfalls

- The ARFI (Acoustic Radiation Force Impulse) pulse attenuates at greater depths
  - This becomes more of an issue when patients have more than 2cm of subcutaneous fat
- Attenuation is greater in a patient with cirrhosis because the liver is stiffer
- Measurements taken while the patient is breathing are inaccurate and will not produce a diagnostic study

Normal Measurements

Structure:	Abbreviation/Acronym:	Measurements:
Interquartile Range/Median	IQR/M	<30% or <0.30
Liver	LIV	<18cm
Meta-analysis of histological data in viral hepatitis	METAVIR	~Look at chart below~
Main Portal Vein	MPV	<13mm Hepatopetal flow (red)

METAVIR

Score:	cm/s:	kPa:	Fibrosis:
F0	<1.35	<5.7	None
F1	1.35-1.66	5.7-8.29	Normal-Mid
F2	1.66-1.77	8.29-9.40	Mid-Moderate
F3	1.77-1.99	9.40-11.9	Moderate-Severe
F4	>1.99	>11.9	Cirrhosis

Notes!

There are a couple of things to keep in mind while doing these studies. The first thing is that elastography exams measure liver stiffness, not fibrosis. After calculating the liver stiffness, we can then determine liver fibrosis. Another important thing to note is that depending on where you work, your department or rads may use either kPa or cm/s. However, cm/s is now becoming more commonly used. I have included both measurements in the chart above.

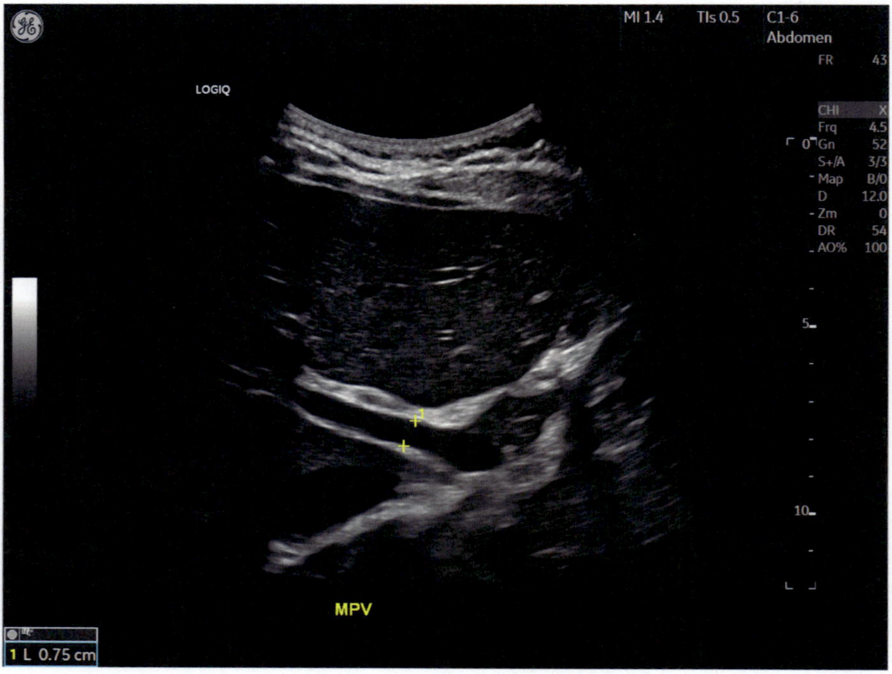

Main portal vein with measurement

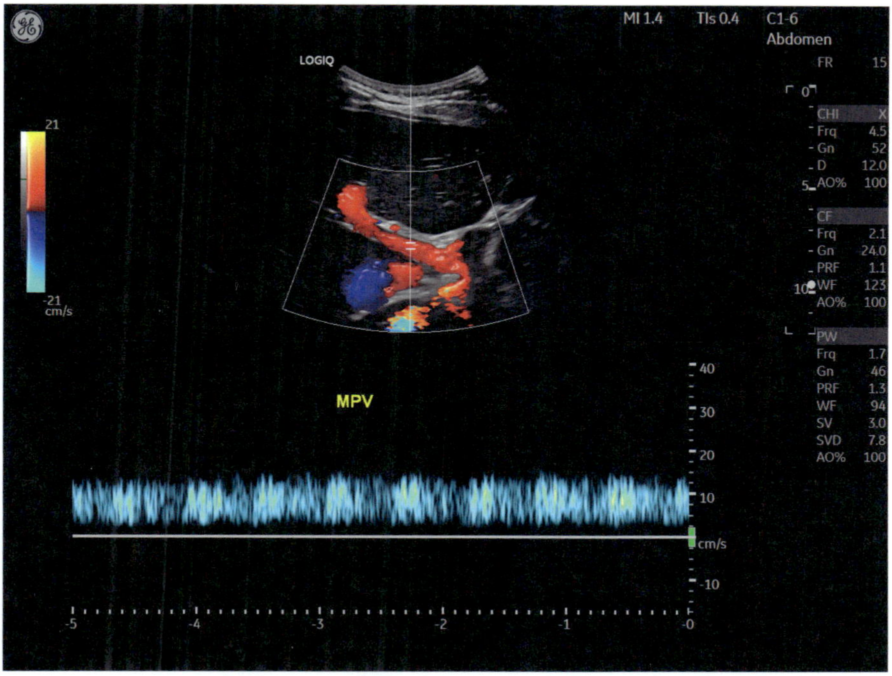

Main portal vein evaluated with color and spectral Doppler

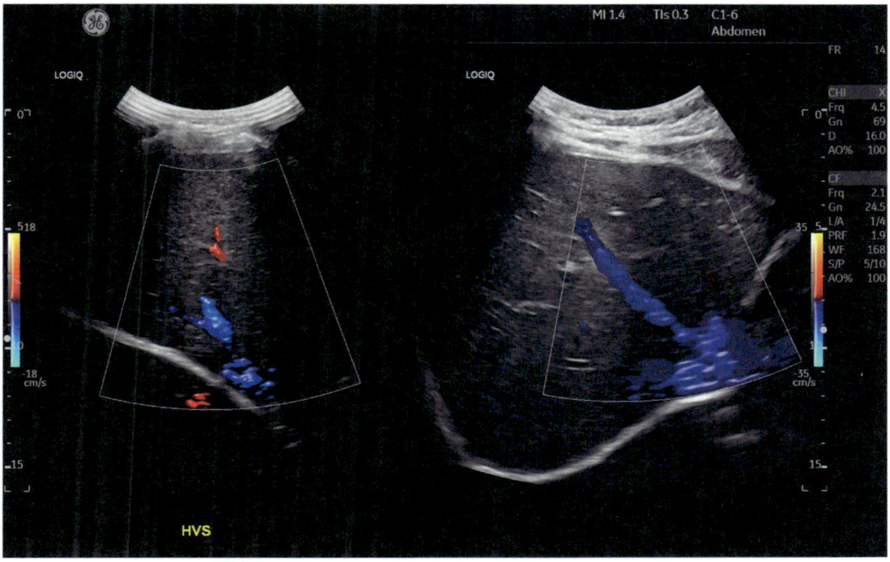

Hepatic veins evaluated with color Doppler

Protocols

Liver Elastography:

1. SAG Liver
   a. 2D: Subcostal/Intercostal
   b. Measurements: L (with RK in the image)
2. TRV Liver
   a. 2D: Subcostal/Intercostal
3. MPV
   a. 2D
   b. Measurements: AP
   c. Color Doppler (normal flow is hepatopetal - red)
   d. Spectral Doppler (normal waveform is above the baseline
4. HVs
   a. Color Doppler (normal flow is hepatofugal - blue)
5. 12 Elastography Samples

Document any liver pathology prior to doing your elastography samples

The amount of elastography samples you take will vary depending on where you work

Notes

Notes

Notes

4

Obstetrics

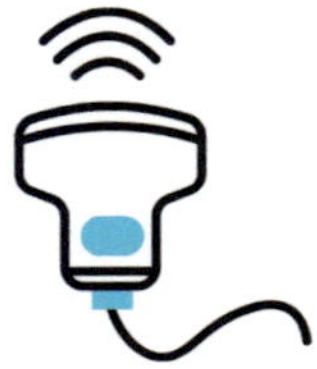

Patient Exam and Prep

For the 1st trimester, anatomy, and viability exams, the patient will need to come with a full bladder. The reason for this is because we want to use the bladder as a window to visualize the cervix and ovaries. For the other exams, no patient prep is needed.

Transducers Used

- Curvilinear C1-6
- Transvaginal transducer IC5-9 (for 1st trimester, viabilities, or cervical exams)

Labs

- AFP
- hCG: >25 = pregnant

For the following protocols, you can acquire the images in any order you would like. Babies move around a lot and may be in inadequate positions for imaging certain things. Therefore, it is ok to skip something and come back to it later on.

1st Trimester

Exam Indications

- Dating
- Viability / pain / vaginal bleeding
- History of previous miscarriages / high risk

Protocol

1. UT
2. CX
3. Ovaries + CL (corpus luteum) + adnexas
4. GS (gestational sac)
5. YS (yolk sac)
6. FP (fetal pole) / CRL (crown rump length)
7. FHR (fetal heart rate)
8. Early placenta (if there is one)

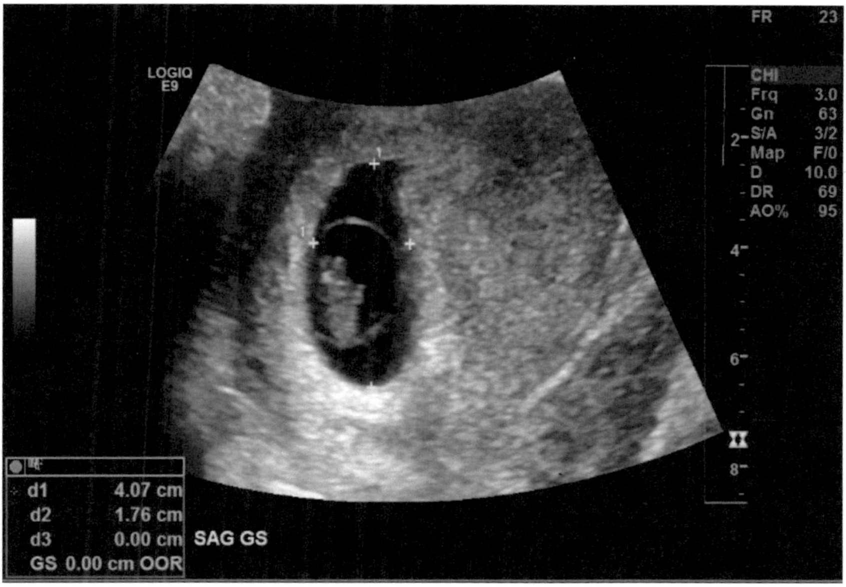

SAG gestational sac measurements

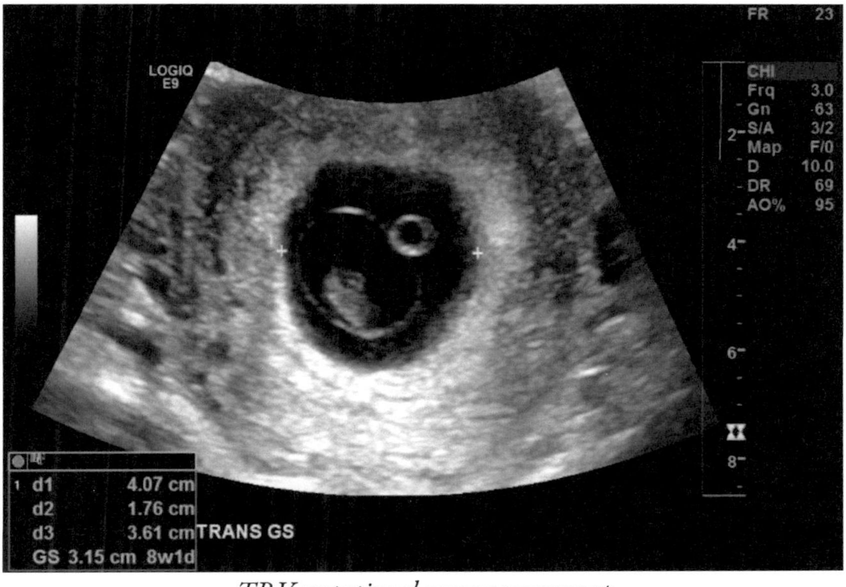

TRV gestational sac measurement

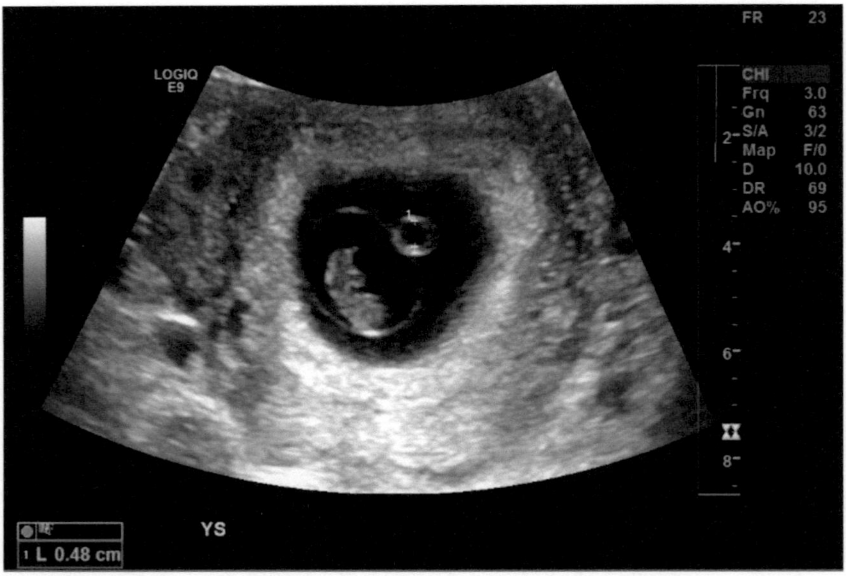

Yolk sac measurement. Measure inner to inner wall in AP

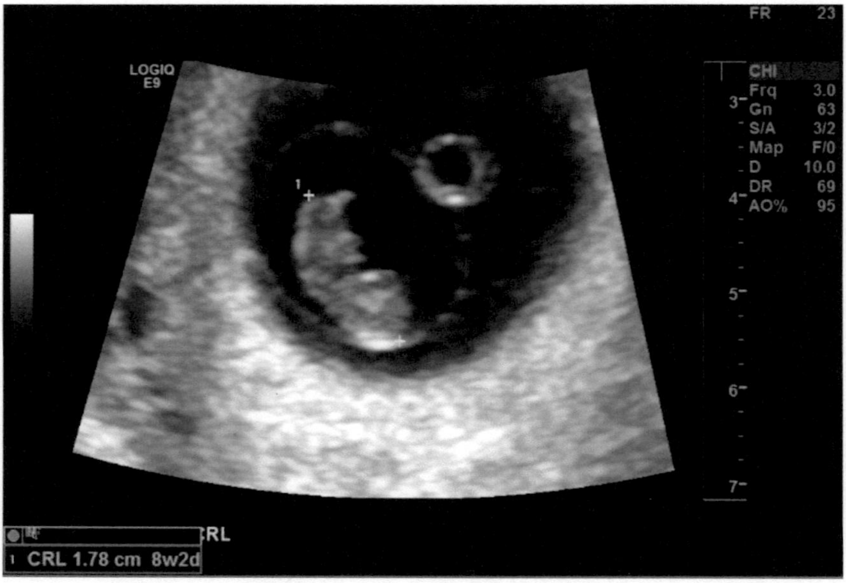

Crown rump length measurement

20-Week Fetal Anatomy

Exam Indications

Normal 20-week anatomy. We want to make sure the baby is healthy and does not have any chromosomal anomalies or congenital defects.

Protocol

Notes!

MFM has many other images that need to be taken for their protocol that are not listed below. In a general lab, we don't normally take those MFM images for our anatomy protocol.

1. CX
2. Fetal position
3. Placenta
4. PCI (placental cord insertion)
5. AFI or MVP (main verticle pocket)
6. HC + BPD
7. Brain structures
    a. Thalamus
    b. CSP (Cavum Septum Pellucidum)

c. Lateral ventricles + choroid plexus

d. Cerebellum

e. Posterior fossa

f. Falx

g. Cisterna magna

h. Nuchal fold

8. Orbits + lenses

9. N/L (nose/lips) + palate

10. Profile + NB (nasal bone)

11. Heart views

a. 4-CH

b. RVOT

c. LVOT

d. AO arch

12. AC

13. Stomach

14. Kidneys

15. ACI (abdominal cord insertion)

16. BL

17. Sex of the fetus

18. LE bones

    a. Femur + FL

    b. Tibia + Fibula

    c. Feet

19. UE bones

    a. Humerus

    b. Radial + Ulnar

    c. Hands

20. Spine

    a. Cervical

    b. Thoracic

    c. Lumbar

    d. Sacral

21. Chest / abdominal wall contour

22. Diaphragm

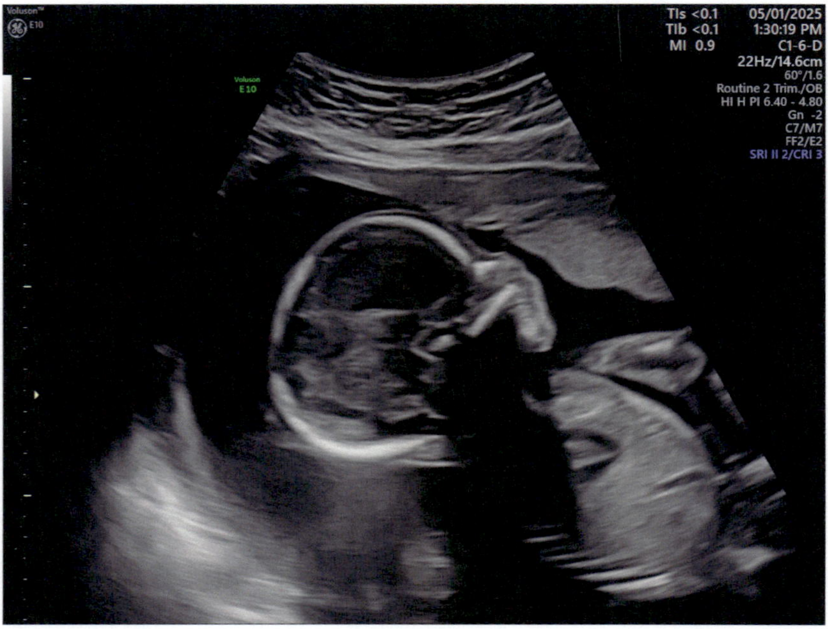

Profile

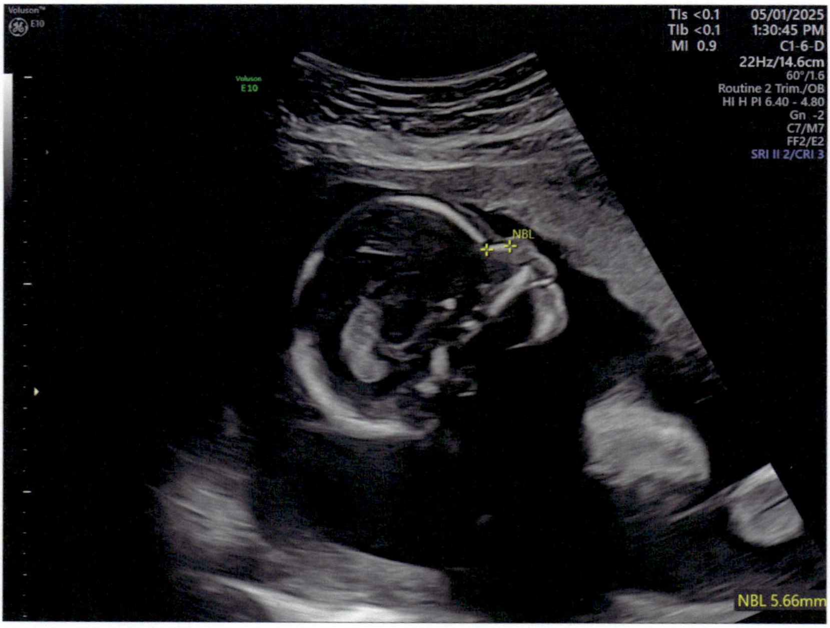

Nasal bone measurement

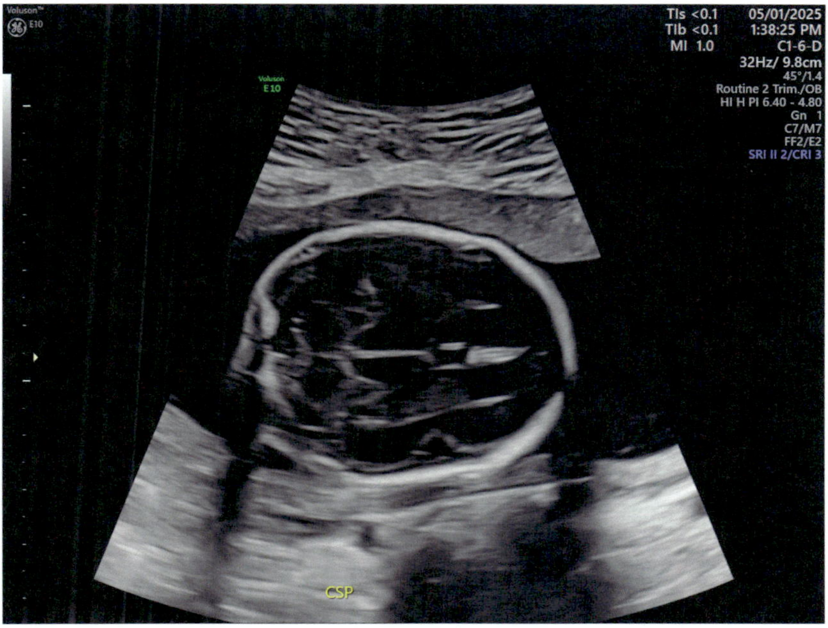

Brain image showing the thalamus and CSP

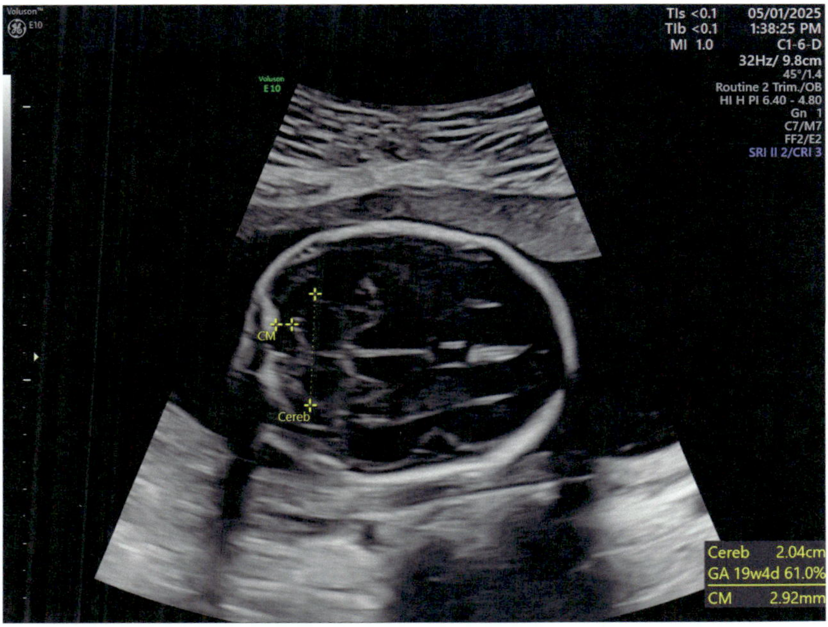

Brain image demonstrating the cerebellum and cisterna magna measurements

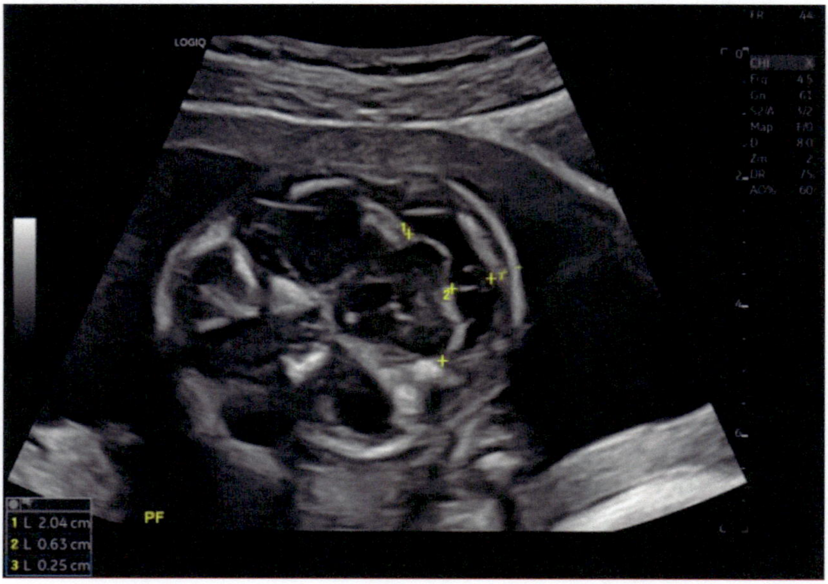

Brain image demonstrating the cerebellum and cisterna magna measurements

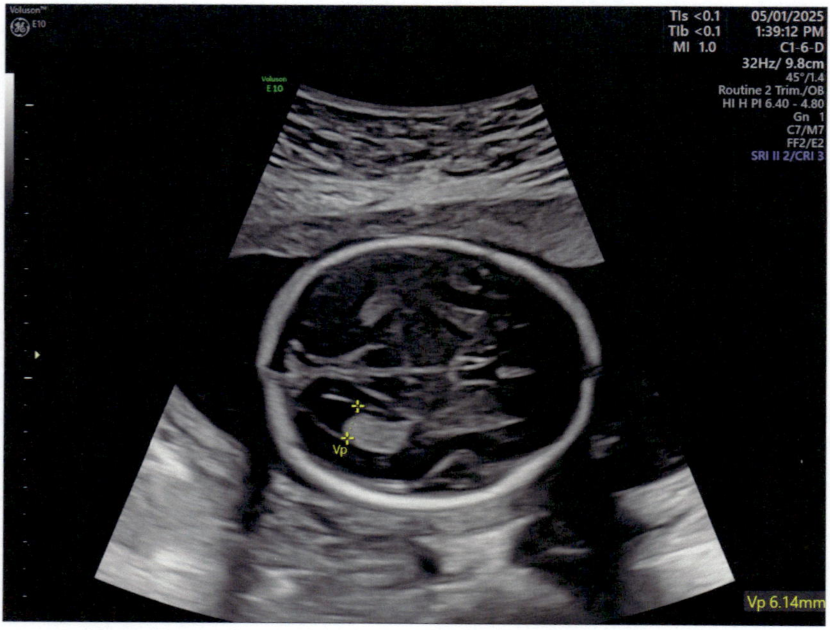

Brain image demonstrating the lateral ventricle measurement

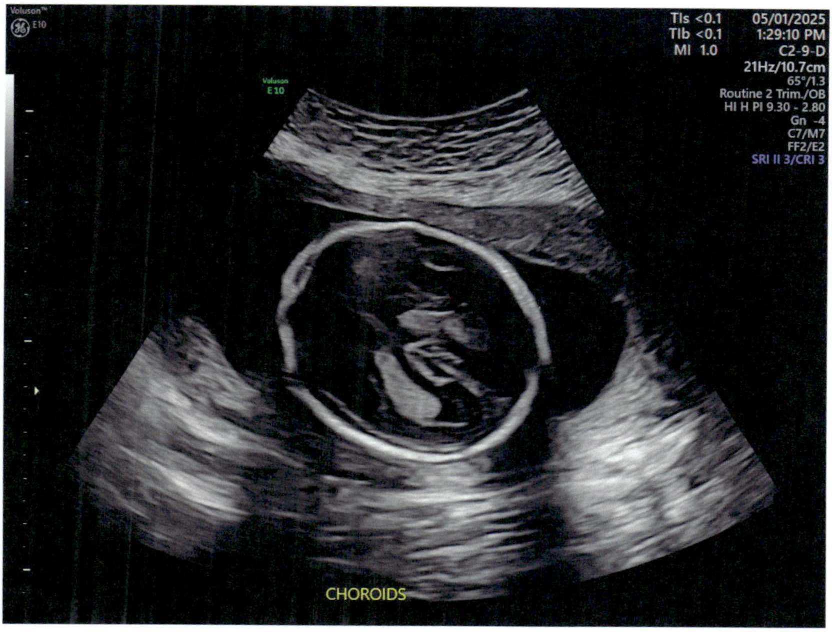

Brain image showing the choroid plexus

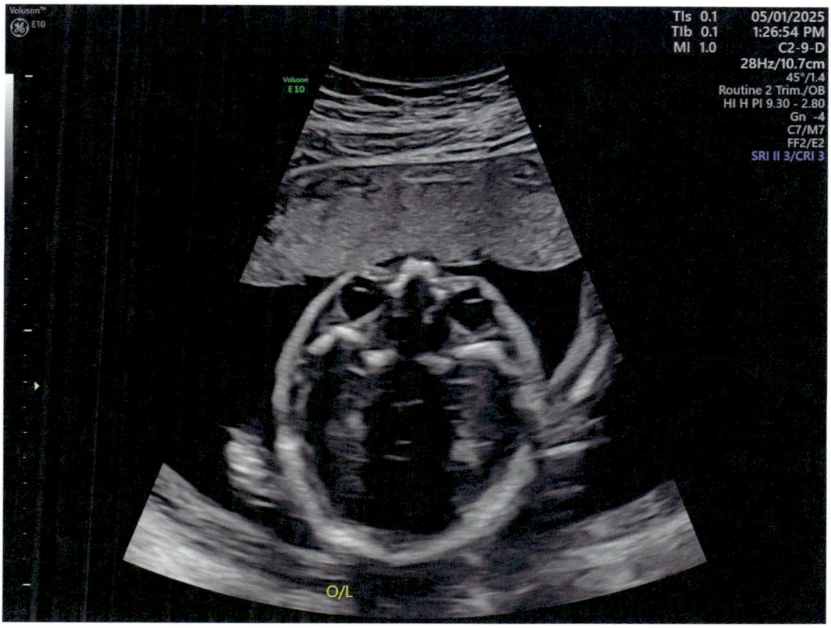

Orbits and lenses

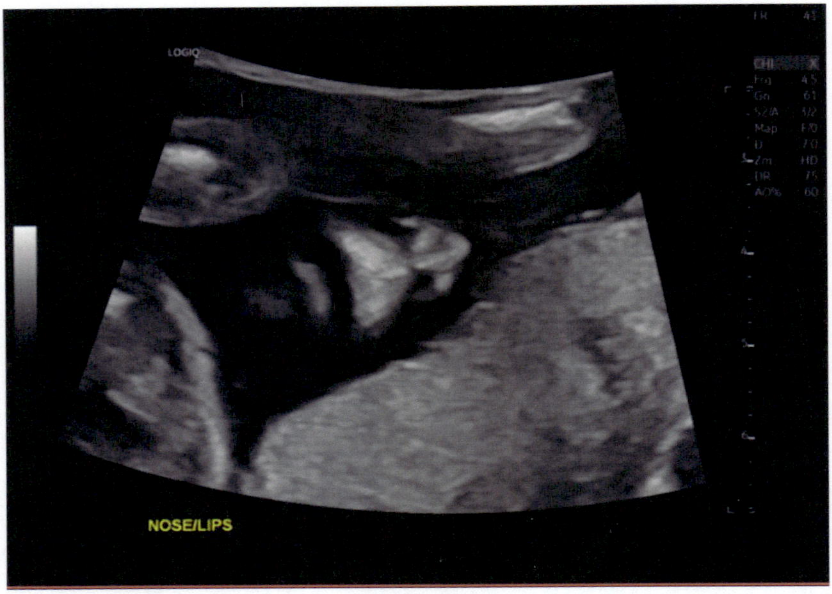

Nose and lips

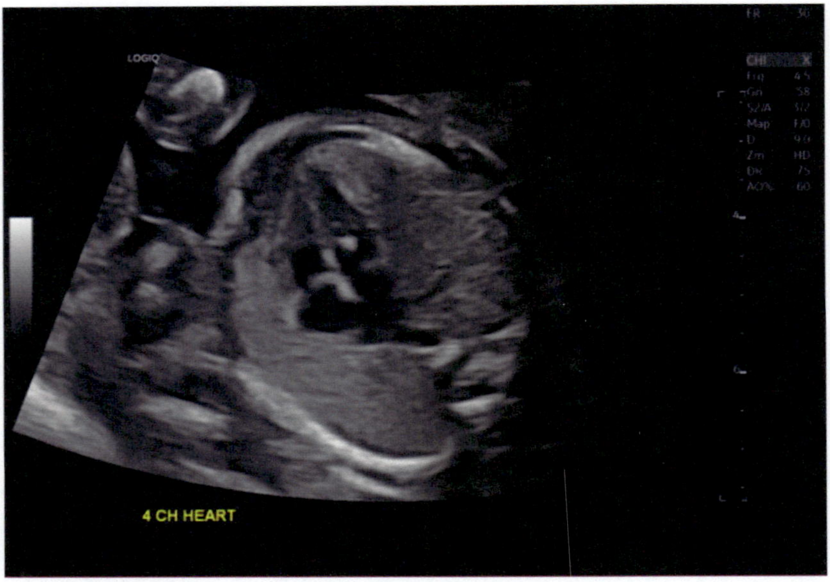

4-champer heart

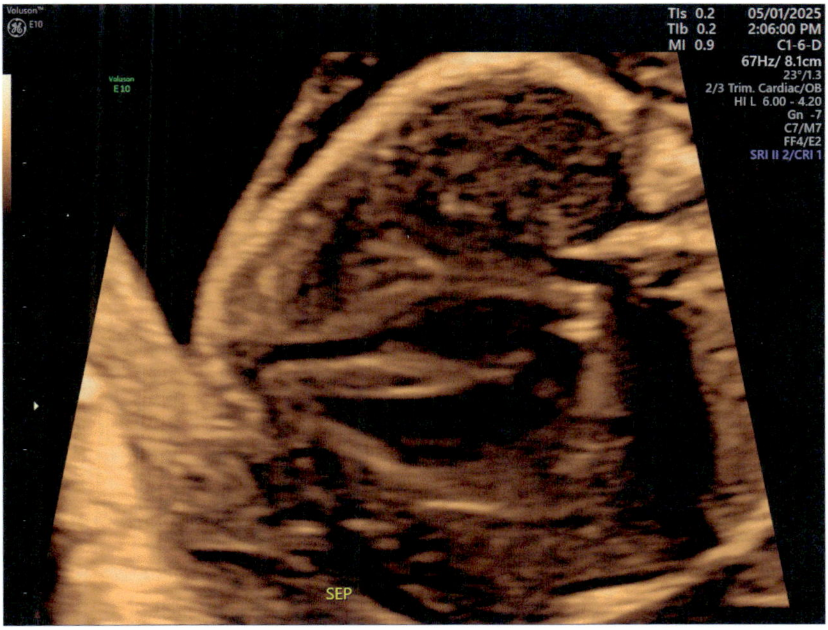

4-chamber heart image showing an intact and normal septum

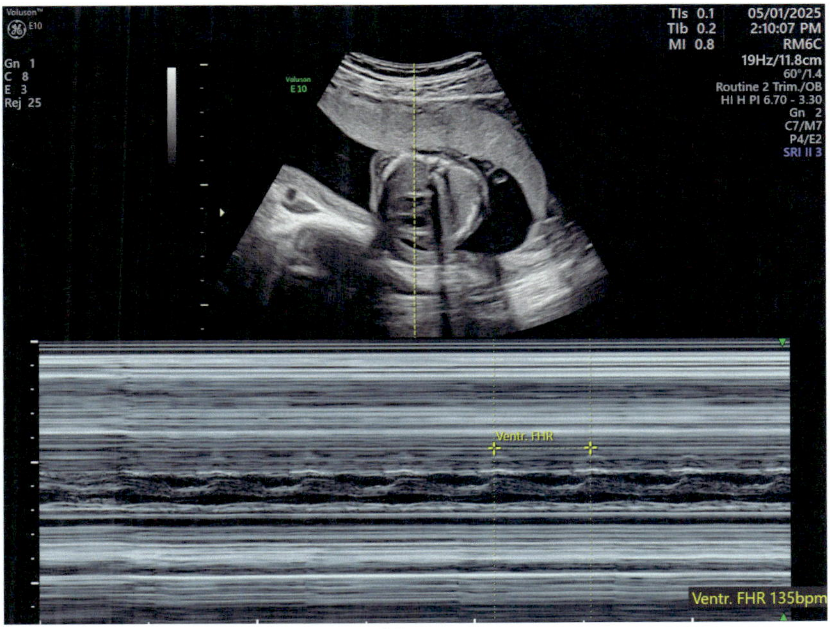

Fetal heart rate

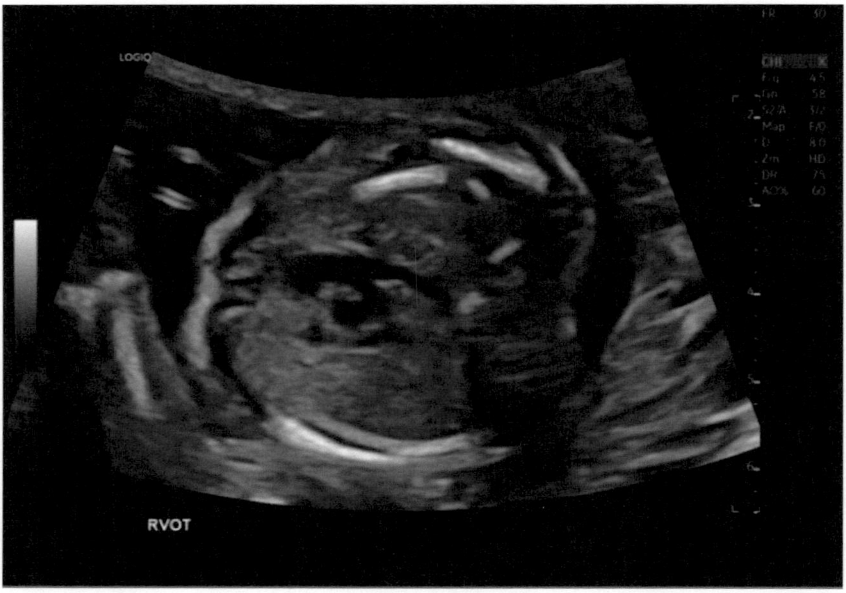

RVOT heart view

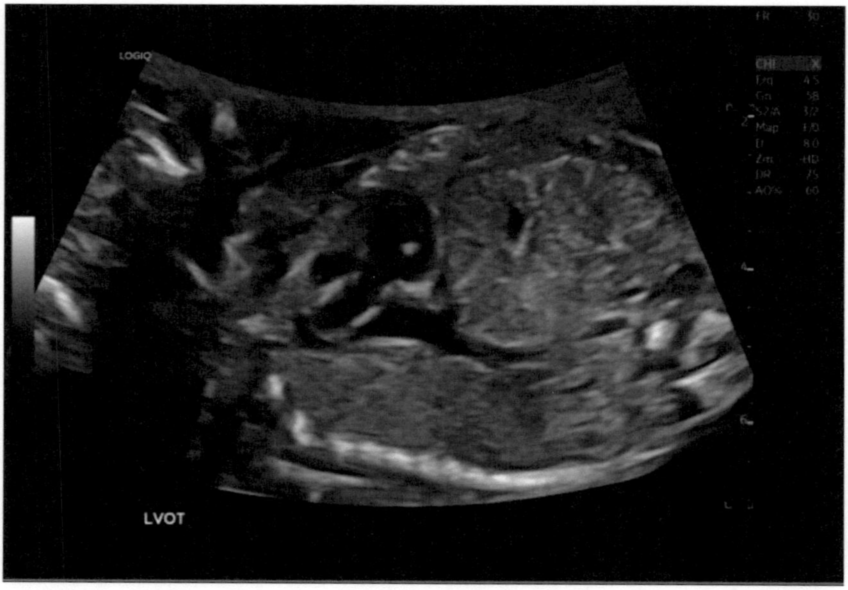

LVOT heart view

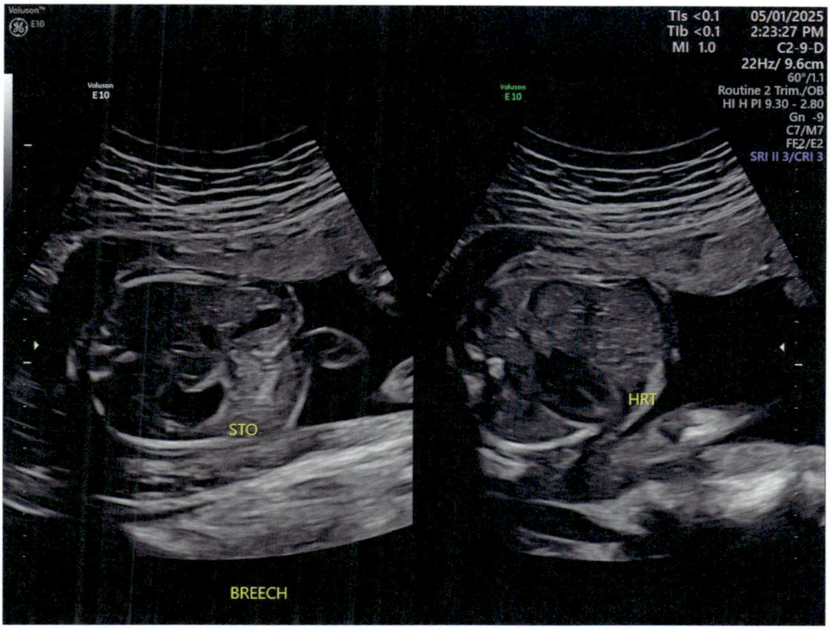

Image demonstrating organ situs solitus (normal organ locations)

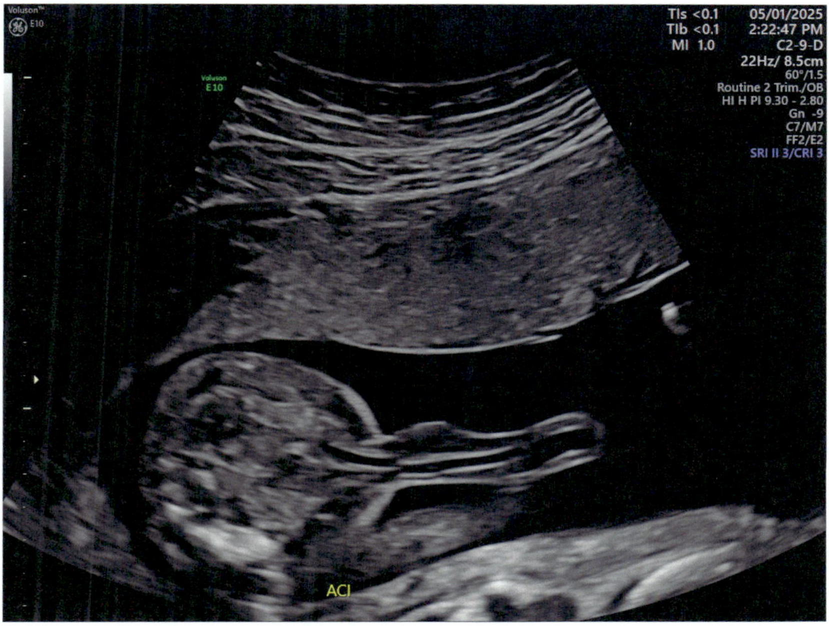

Abdominal cord insertion

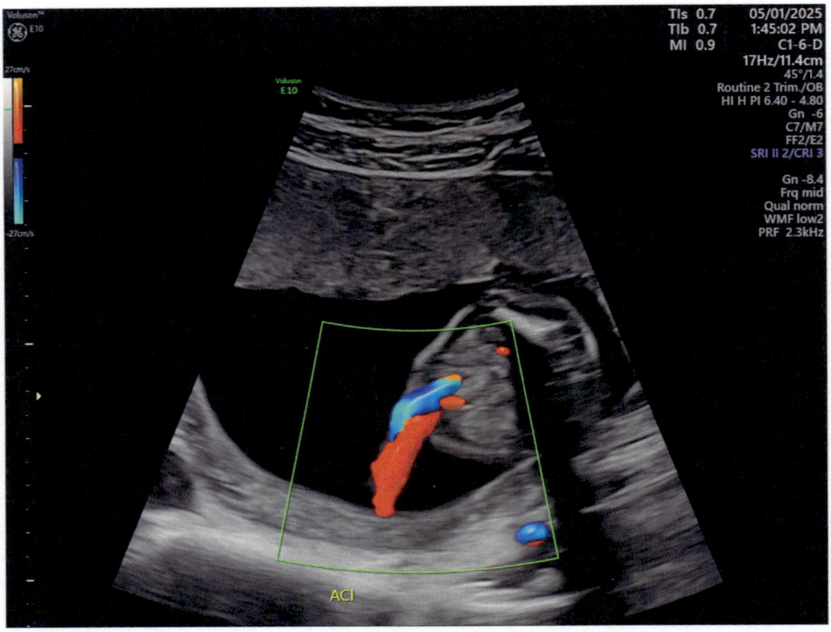

Abdominal cord insertion evaluated with color Doppler

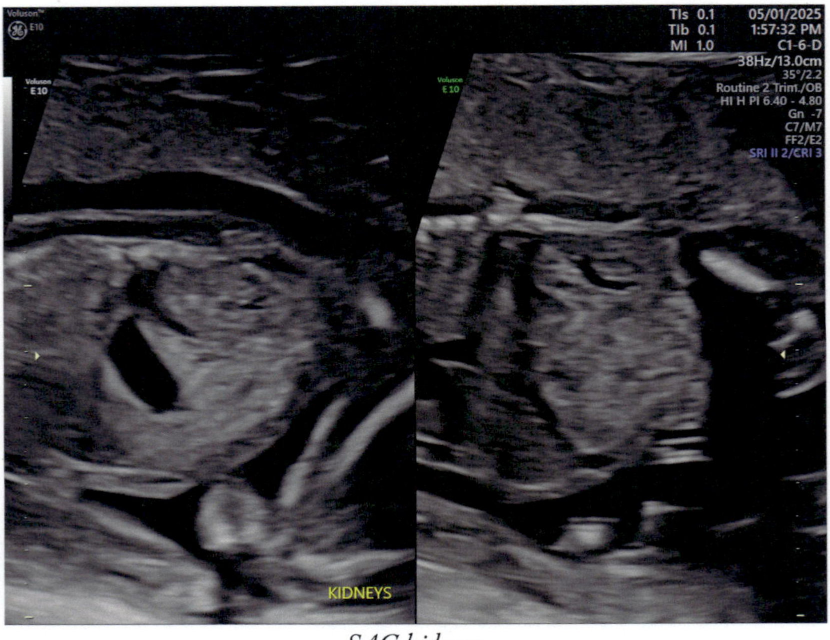

SAG kidneys

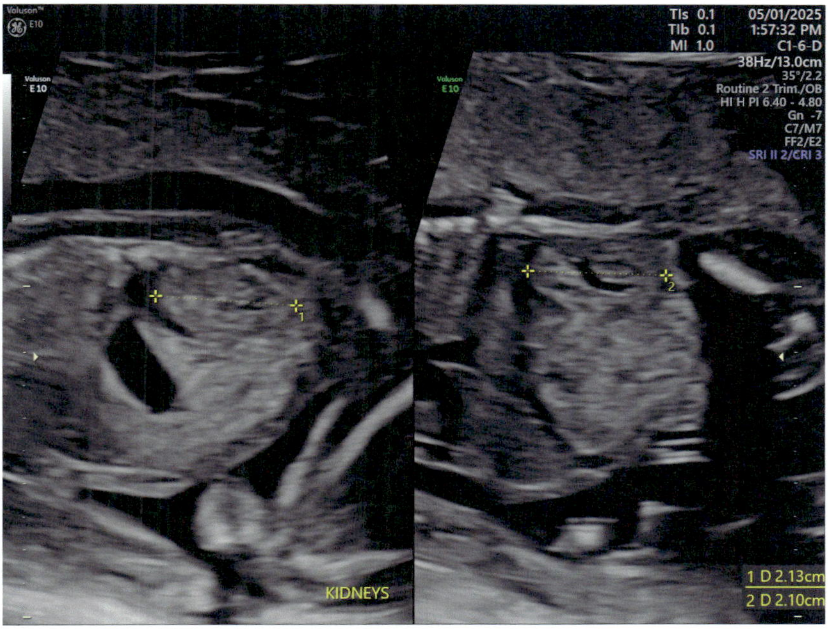

SAG kidneys with measurements

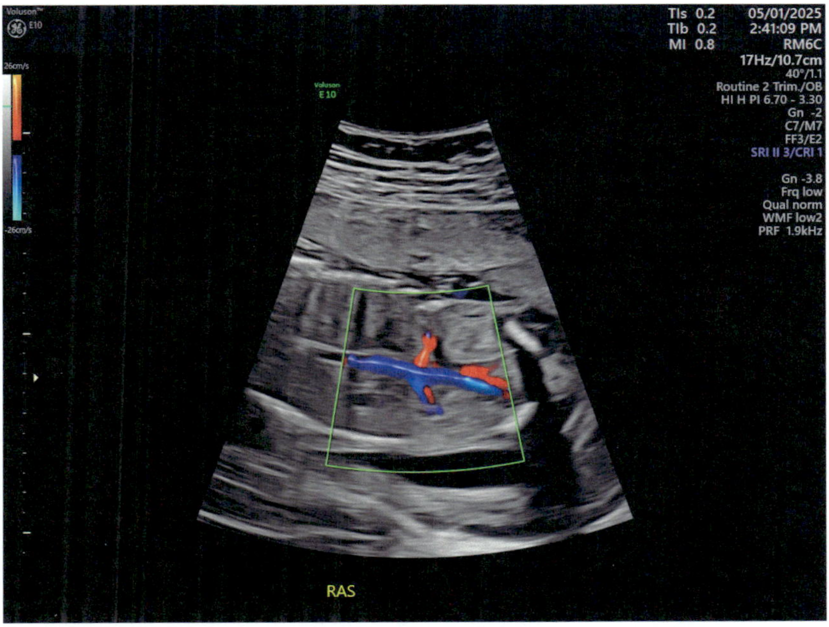

Kidneys evaluated with color Doppler showing the renal arteries

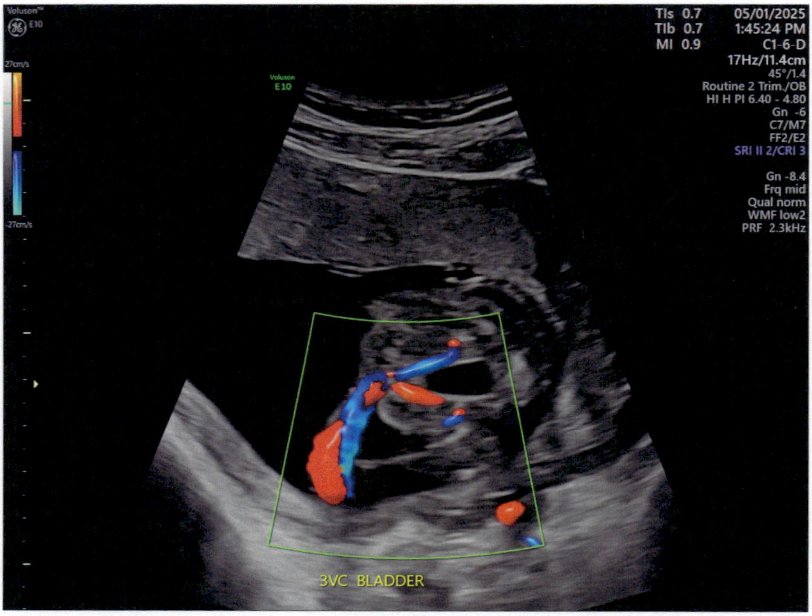

Bladder and 3 vessel cord evaluated with color Doppler

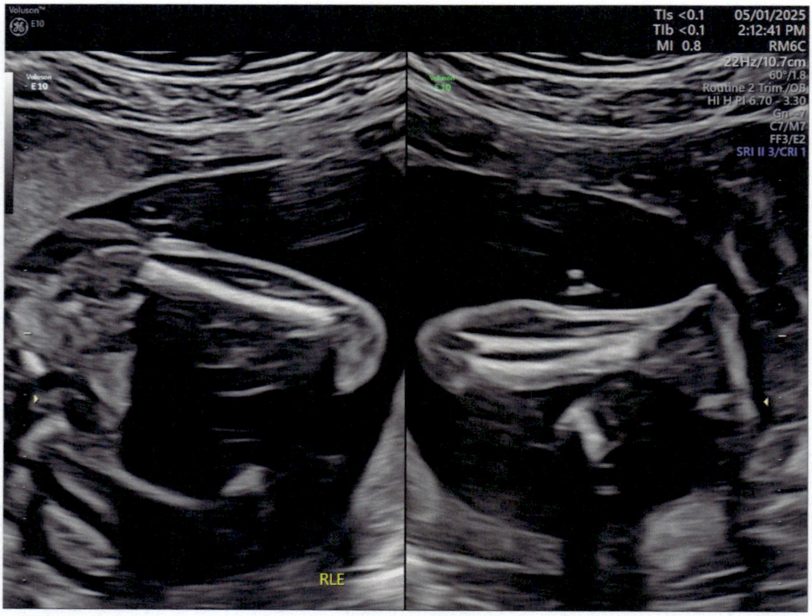

Right lower extremity image showing the femur bone on the left and the tibia and fibula bones on the right

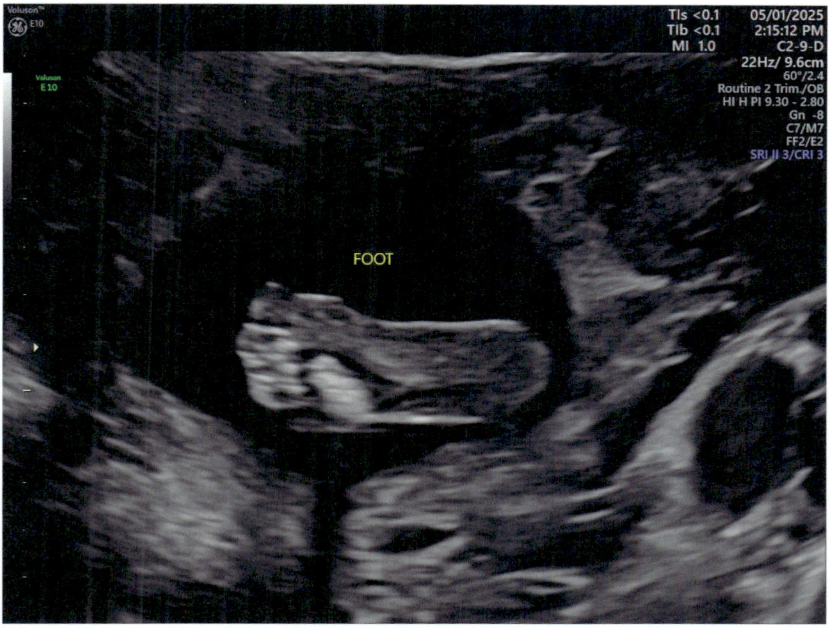

Foot

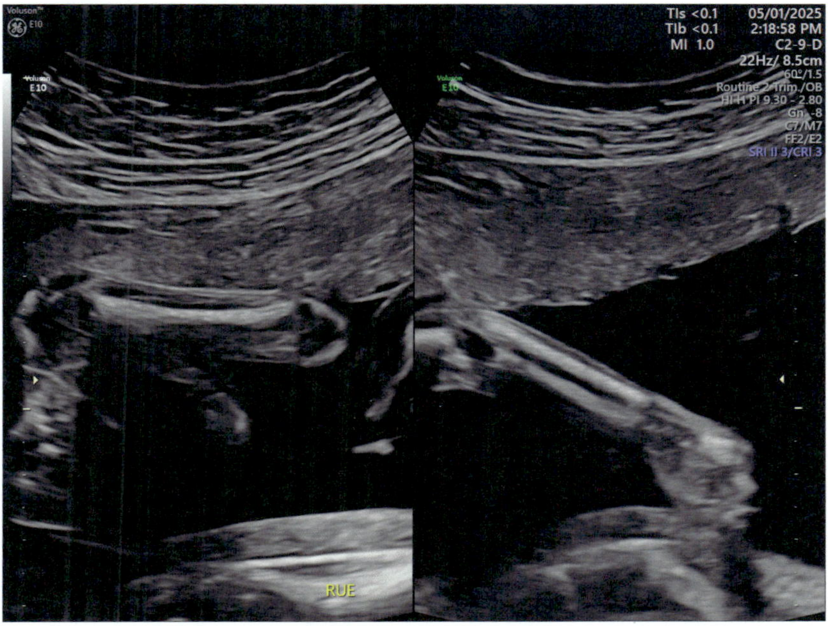

Right upper extremity image showing the humerus bone on the left and the radial and ulnar bones on the right

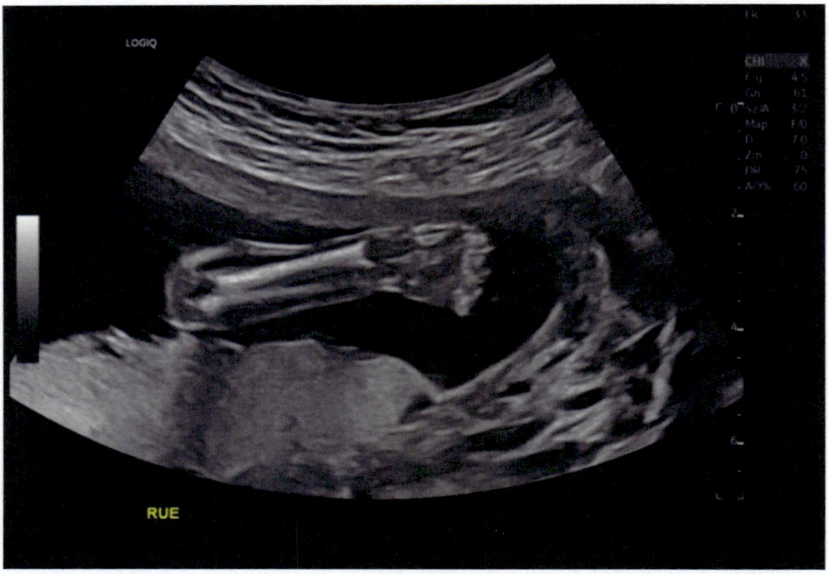

Hand

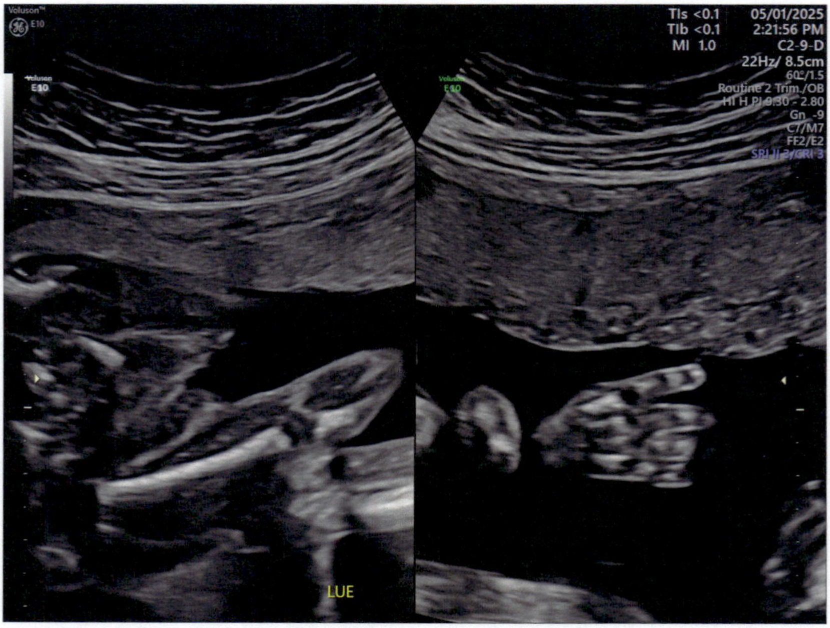

Left upper extremity + hand

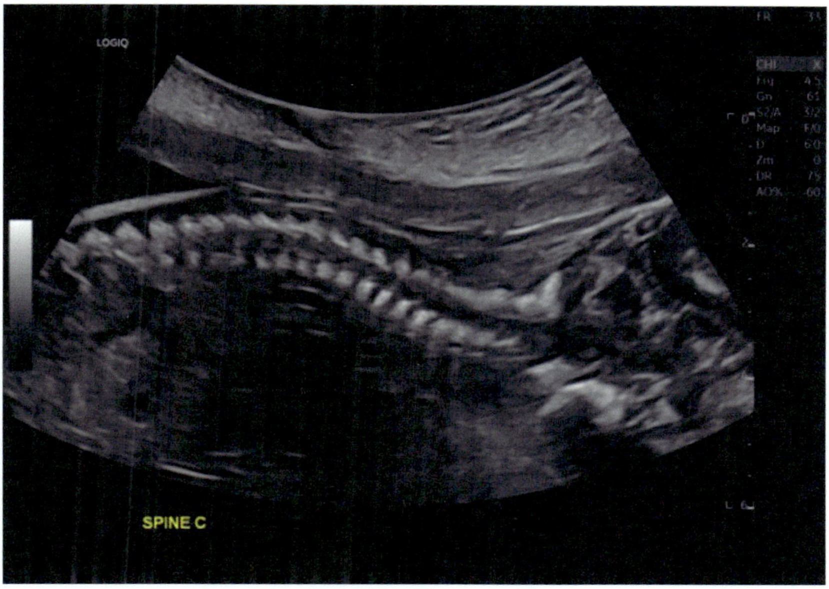

Cervical spine

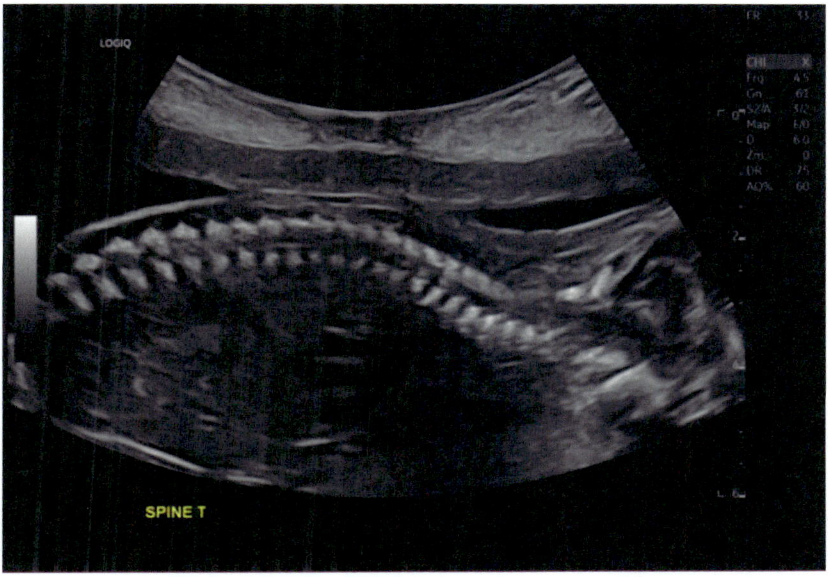

Thoracic spine

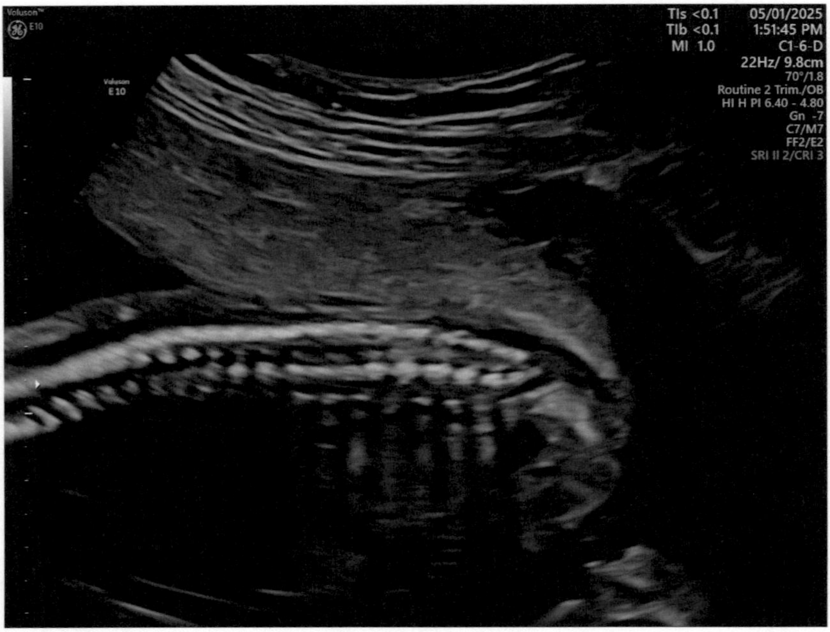

Lumbar + sacral spine

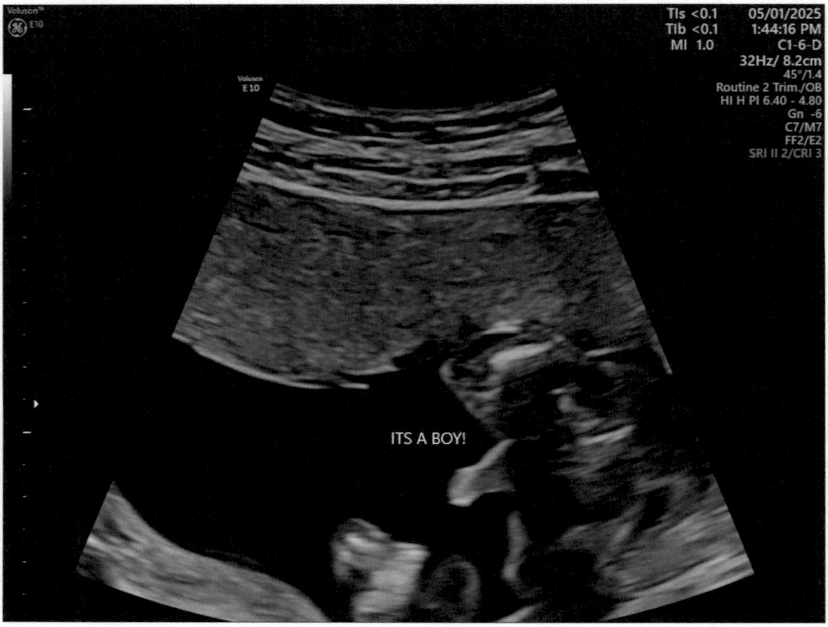

Male fetus

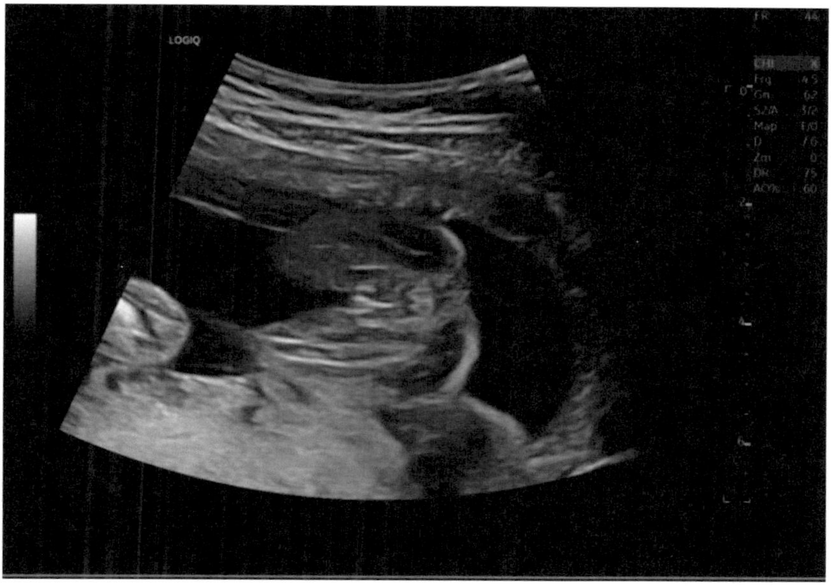

Female fetus

Additional MFM images may include:

1. Head + Neck:
   a. Maxilla
   b. Mandible
   c. Tongue
   d. Ears
2. Fetal Heart:
   a. 3VV (3 Vessel View)
   b. 3VT (3 Vessel Trachea)

c. Ductal Arch

d. IVC + SVC

3. Abdomen:

a. Liver

b. Small + Large Bowel

c. Adrenal Glands

d. GB

e. Spleen

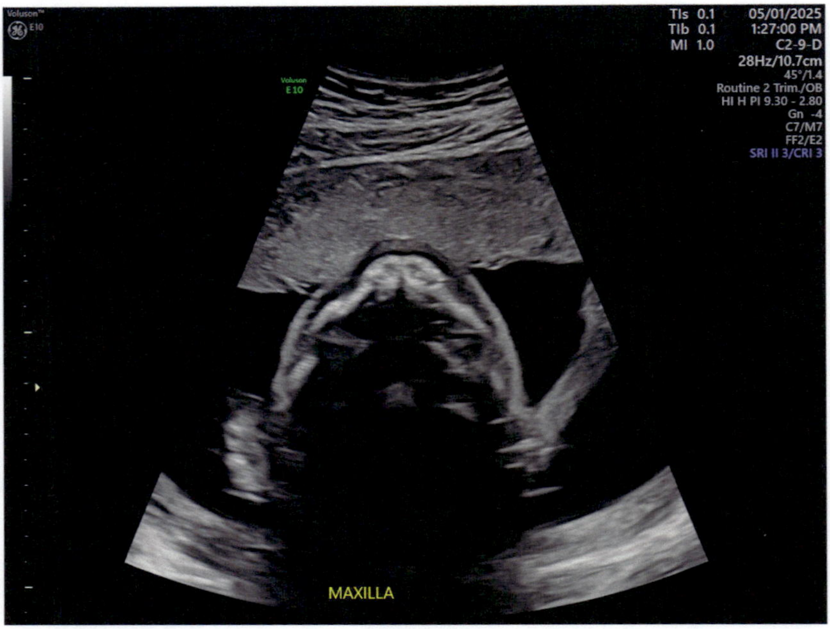

Maxilla

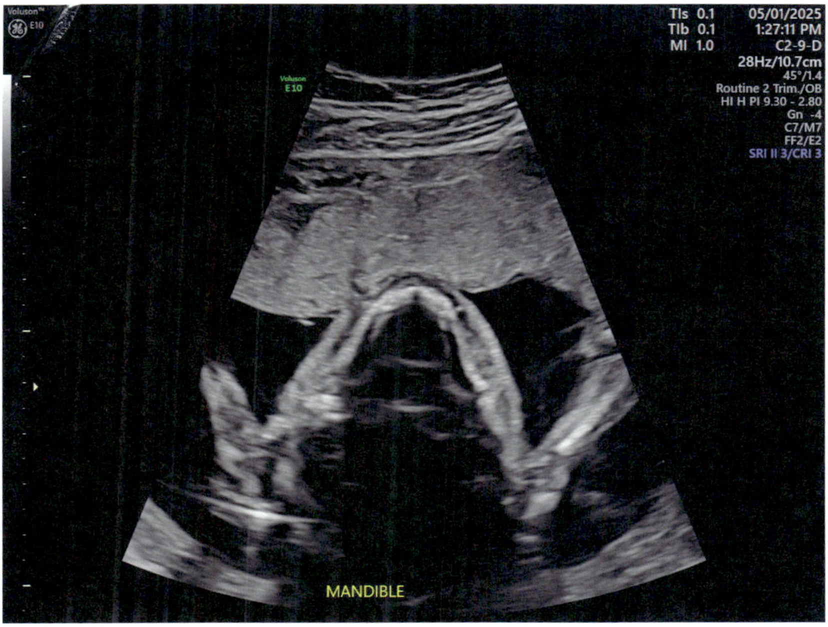

Mandible

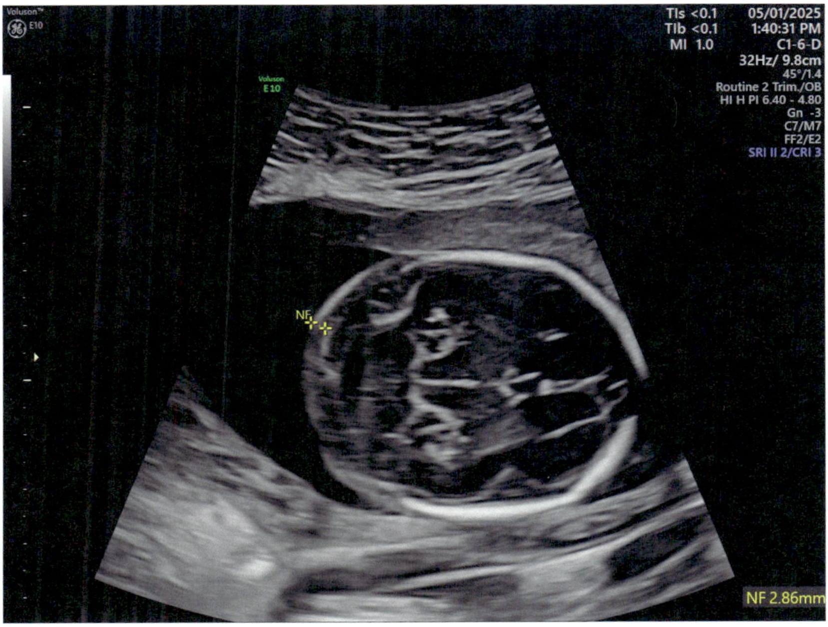

Brain image demonstrating the nuchal fold measurement

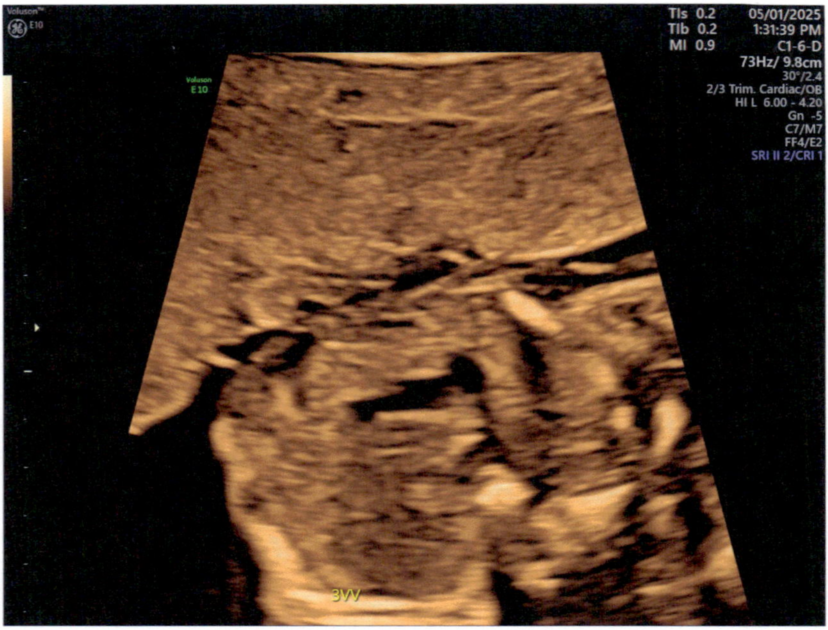

Fetal heart 3 vessel view

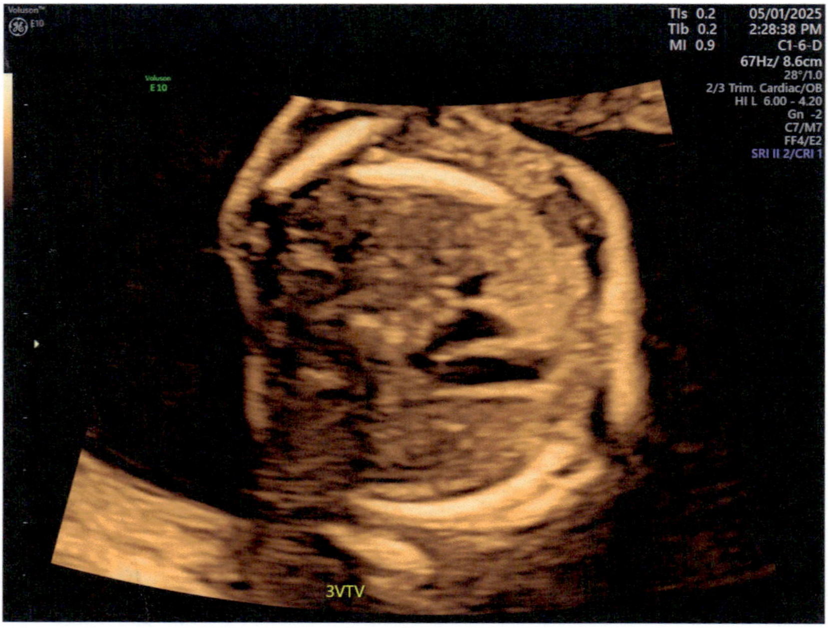

3-vessel trachea heart view

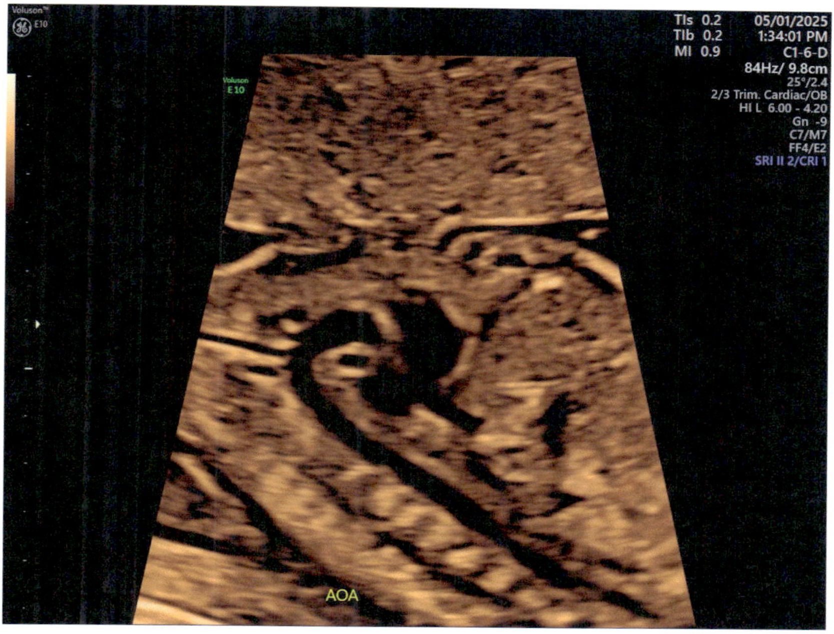

Aortic arch heart view

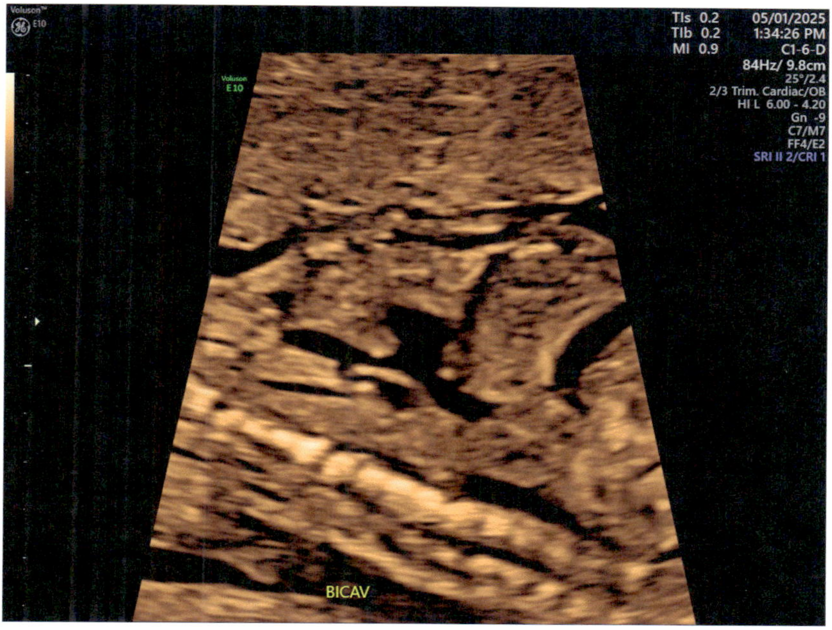

Bicaval heart view

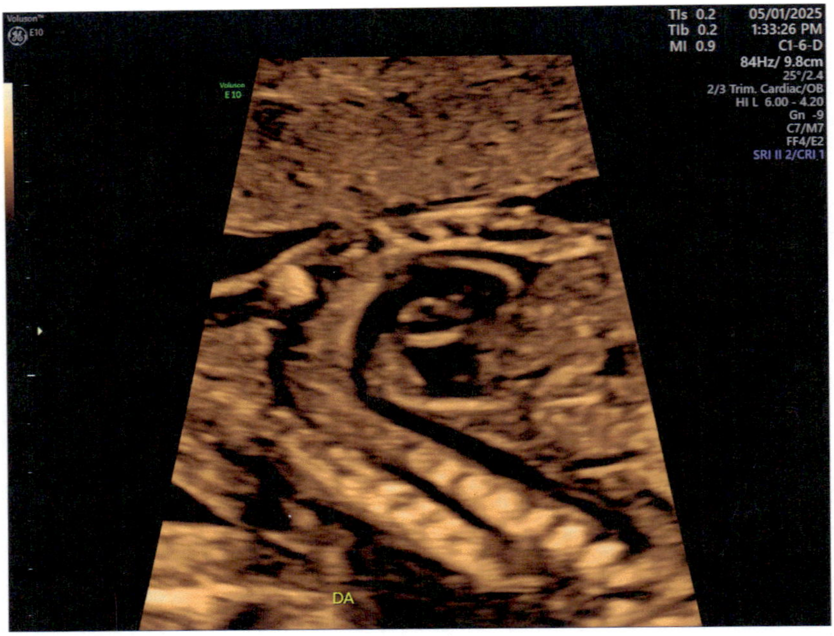

Ductal arch view

AFI

Exam Indications

- High risk
- Oligohydramnios
- Polyhydramnios
- Suspected anhydramnios

Protocol

Notes!

The AFI varies greatly depending on what trimester the patient is in and is affected by many fetal conditions.

1. CX
2. Fetal position
3. Placenta
4. FHR
5. Fluid-filled structures
    a. Stomach
    b. Kidneys

c. BL

6. MVP in each of the 4 quadrants calculating an AFI. (Only calculate an AFI if the fetus is over 28 weeks. If the fetus is under 28 weeks, only do an MVP and not an AFI).

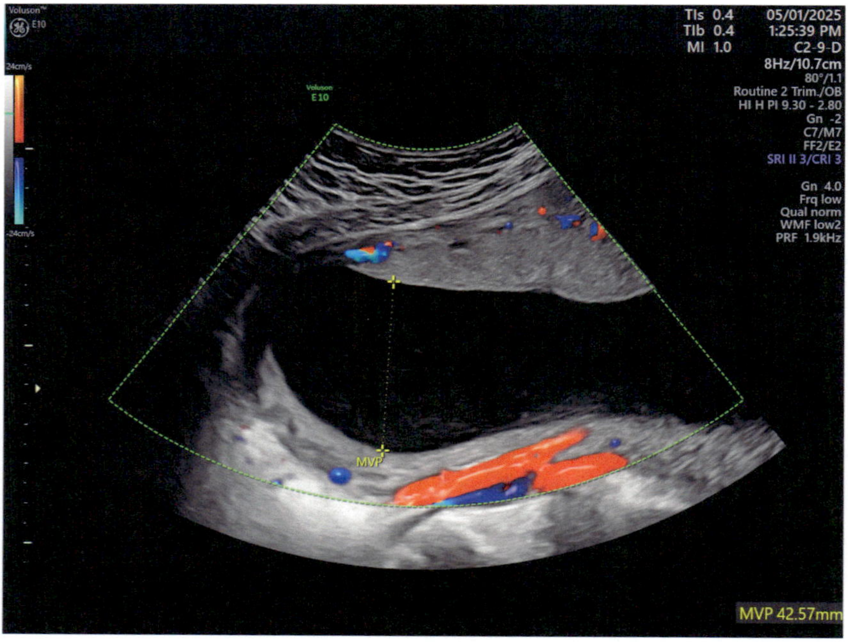

Main vertical pocket measurement

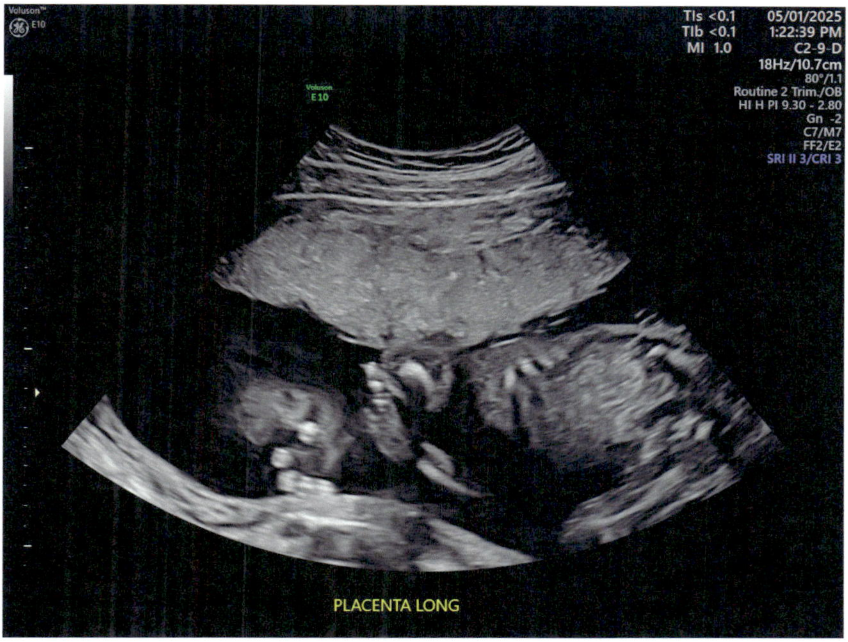

Anterior SAG placenta

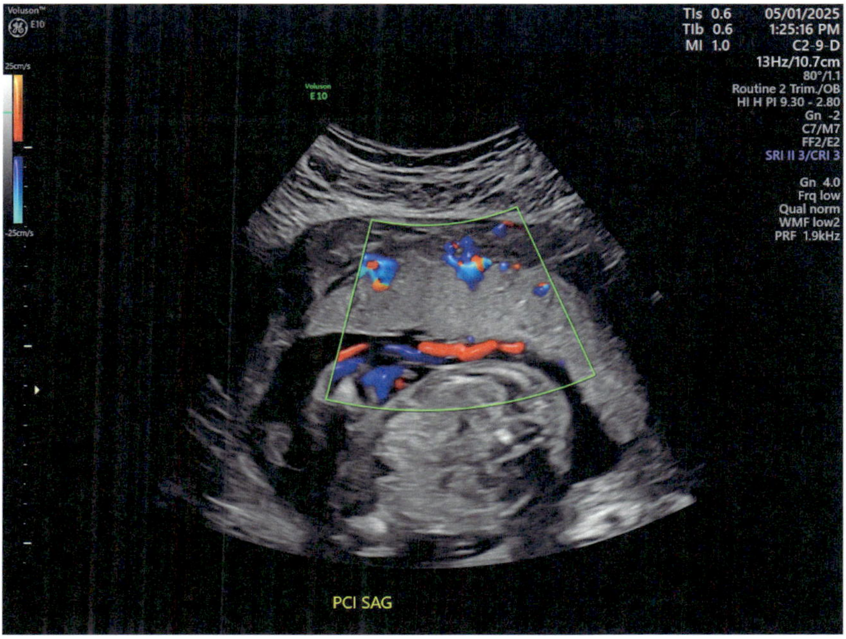

Placenta cord insertion

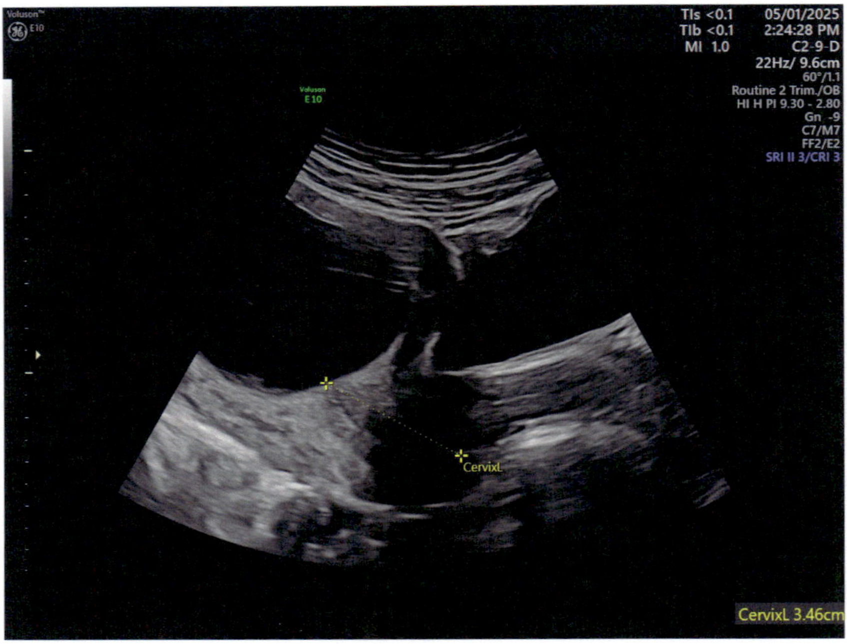

Cervical measurement

BPP

Exam Indications

- High risk
    - HTN
    - Gestational diabetes
    - AMA (advanced maternal age)
    - Post-dates
    - Growth restriction
- Decreased fetal movement

Protocol

Notes!

The fetus is scored on a scale out of 8, with each parameter getting a score of either 0 or 2. There is NO such thing as a score of 1. The four parameters are

1. Breathing motion
2. Gross fetal movement
3. Fetal Tone
4. AFI

If the baby presents with all 4 things, they will score an 8 out of 8. If the baby presents with everything except breathing motion, then the baby will score a 6 out of 8.

The exam has a maximum time limit of 30 minutes to acquire all images, then the test is done. You are not allowed to scan for more than 30 minutes.

A quick tip on getting breathing motion. I always check for breathing motion first. For some reason, babies tend to do it at the beginning of the exam rather than later. At least that is what I have found.

1. CX
2. Fetal position
3. Placenta
4. FHR
5. Fluid-filled structures
    a. Stomach
    b. Kidneys
    c. BL
6. Gross fetal movement (big body movements) – 2pts
7. Fetal tone (ex: flexion of the legs and arms) – 2pts
8. Breathing (motion of the diaphragm) – 2pts
9. AFI – 2pts

Fetal Growth

Exam Indications

- Fetus is not measuring accurately for dates
- Fetus is over 40 weeks GA
- High risk
    - Gestational diabetes
    - HTN
    - AMA
    - Teen pregnancy
    - Drug use

Protocol

1. CX
2. Fetal position
3. Placenta
4. FHR
5. Fluid-filled structures
    a. Stomach

b. Kidneys

c. BL

6. AFI or MVP

7. BPD (biparietal diameter)

   a. Landmarks for this image are the thalamus and CSP. Don't have the cerebellum in view, otherwise you are off-axis

8. HC (head circumference)

   a. Landmarks for this image are the same as the BPD and will be taken in the same image as the BPD

9. AC (abdominal circumference)

   a. Landmarks for this image include the stomach, umbilical vein, and portal sinus

10. FL (femur length)

    a. Measure the most anterior femur

    b. You want the femur to be as flat and parallel to the transducer as possible. Don't measure it at an angle

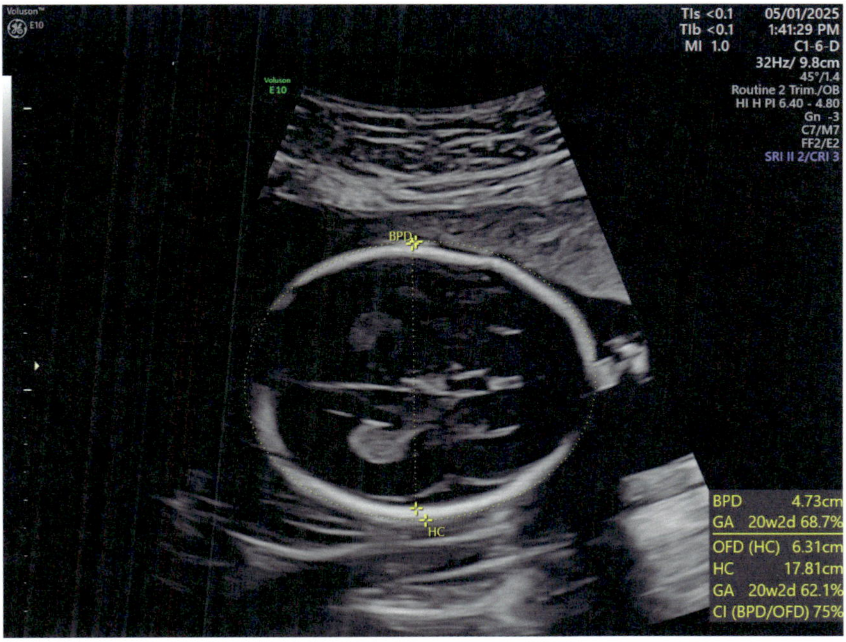

BPD and HC measurements

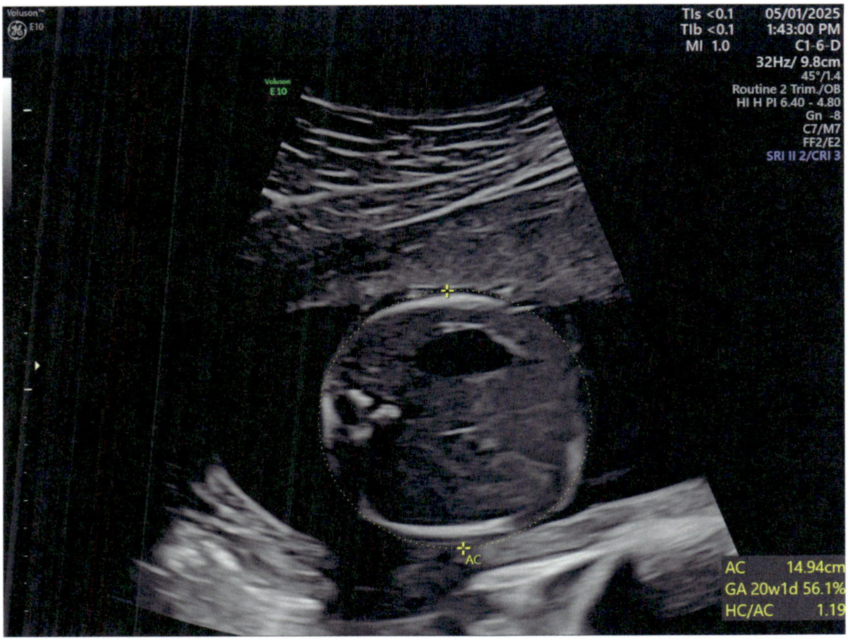

AC measurement

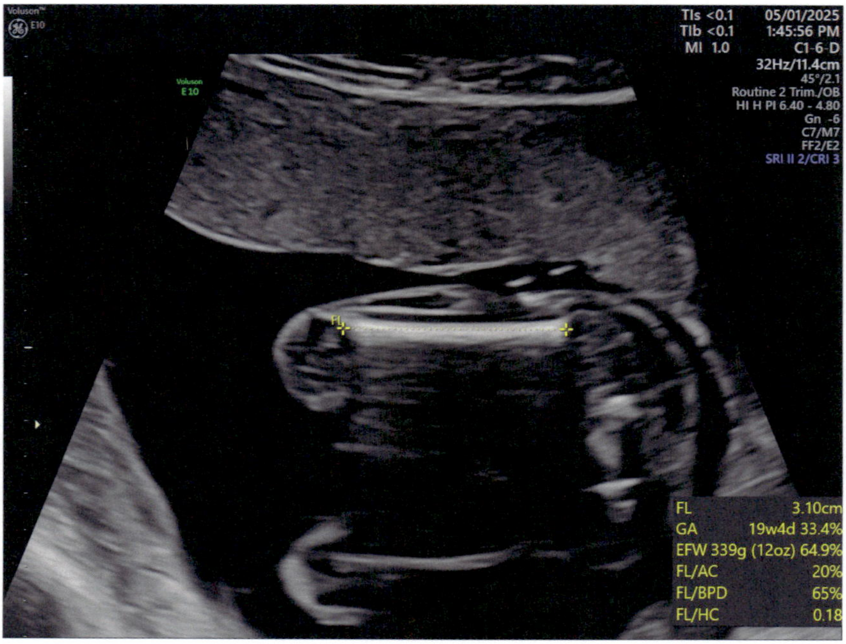

FL measurement

Nuchal Translucency

Exam Indications

- To rule out chromosomal anomalies such as Trisomy 21

Protocol

Notes!

This exam is on a time frame. It can only be performed when the fetus' CRL measures between 45-84mm. This typically translates to a gestational age between 11-13 weeks and 6 days. It CANNOT be performed outside of that time frame.

During this exam the sonographer will perform an early 1st trimester scan while focusing more on what is called the NT (nuchal translucency). This is the fluid-filled space that lies at the back of the neck and is measured by the sonographer. The reason why sonographers measure this space is because a thickened NT can correlate with many types of chromosomal anomalies, such as down syndrome. It can also be an indicator of congenital heart disease, amongst other things.

Patients will then speak with a genetic counselor afterward as this exam is part of the genetic screening process.

1. Complete 1st trimester US
    a. Also show that the heart is inside the chest
2. Choroid plexus

3. Profile + NB

4. Fluid-filled structures

    a. Stomach

    b. BL

5. ACI

6. Upper extremities

7. Lower extremities

8. NT

Viability

Exam Indications

- Trauma
- Px
- VB

Protocol

Notes!

If this is a fetus in the 1st trimester, do a complete 1st trimester exam. If the fetus is in 2nd or 3rd trimester, do parts 2, 4, and 5.

1. CX
2. Placenta (if there is one)
3. FHR
4. MVP or AFI (only if this is a 2nd or 3rd-trimester exam)
5. Fluid-filled structures
    a. Stomach
    b. Kidneys
    c. BL

Normal Measurements

Structure:	Abbreviation/ Acronym:	Measurements:	Notes:
Anhydramnios		0cm or close to that	No fluid or close to having no fluid
Cerebellum	CERE	mm = GA in weeks ex: GA = 19 weeks cere = 19mm *This measurement only works up to 20 weeks GA. After 20 weeks, the cere grows faster and larger than the GA	Both lobes should be symmetric in size and shape
Cervix	CX	≥3cm	Should be closed and no signs of funneling
Cisterna Magna	CM	<10mm	A CSF (cerebrospinal fluid) space located in the PF (posterior fossa)
Cavum Septum Pellucidum	CSP	-	Should always be seen between 18-37 weeks

Normal Measurements Continued

Structure:	Abbreviation/ Acronym:	Measurements:	Notes:
Fetal Heart Rate	FHR	1st Tri: <180bpm 2nd Tri: <150bpm 3rd Tri: <150bmp	FHR decreases over time
Lateral Ventricles	LV or LAT VENTS	<1cm	Contains the choroid plexus
Maximum Vertical Pocket	MVP	>2cm	Amniotic fluid assessment, but measuring the largest pocket (one of the four quadrants) in AP diameter
Nasal Bone	NB	>4mm	-
Nuchal Fold	NF	<5mm	Fluid space between the occipital bone and skin
Nuchal Translucency	NT	Risk of aneuploidy: % <2mm = <1% 3.4mm = 7% 3.5 - 4.4mm = 20% 5.5 - 6.4mm = 50% >8.5mm = 75%	Must be done between 11-13 weeks and 6 days

Normal Measurements Continued

Structure:	Abbreviation/ Acronym:	Measurements:	Notes:
Oligohydramnios	OLIGO	AFI: <5cm MVP: <2cm	Too little amniotic fluid
Placenta Distance from Internal Os	-	>2cm = normal <2cm = low lying	*See chart below for types*
Placenta Cord Insertion from Placenta Edge	PCI	>2cm	*See chart below for types*
Polyhydramnios	POLY	AFI: >24cm MVP: >8cm	Too much amniotic fluid
Yolk Sac	YS	<7mm	Only seen in early 1st trimester

Trimesters:

Trimester:	Abbreviation/Acronym:	Notes:
1st	Tri 1	0-13 weeks
2nd	Tri 2	14-27 weeks
3rd	Tri 3	28-40 weeks

Twins:

Twin Type:	Abbreviation / Acronym:	Notes:
Dichorionic - Diamniotic	Di - Di	2 chorions + 2 amnions
Monochorionic - Diamniotic	Mo - Di	1 chorion + 2 amnions
Monochorionic - Monoamniotic	Mo - Mo	1 chorion + 1 amnion

Placenta Locations:

Placental Location:	Notes:
Anterior	Located along the anterior portion of the uterus
Posterior	Located along the posterior portion of the uterus
Fundal	Located within the uterine fundus
Right / Left Lateral Lying	Located either to the right or left in the uterus – will also be located either anteriorly or posteriorly
Low-Lying	Located within 2cm of the cx internal os
Previa	
Complete	Completely covers the cx internal os
Partial	Covers a portion of the cx internal os
Marginal	The placental edge just reaches the cx internal os, but does not cover any portion of the cx

Types of Cord Insertions

Type:	Notes:
Central	Cord inserts into the placenta centrally or in/near the middle
Lateral	Cord inserts into the placenta laterally >2cm from the placental edge
Marginal	Cord inserts into the placenta <2cm from the placental edge
Velamentous	Cord inserts into the chorio-amniotic membranes, then travels between them (amnion + chorion) to the placenta, leaving the umbilical vessels exposed

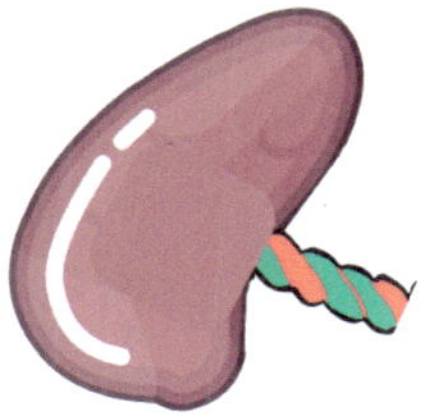

Central

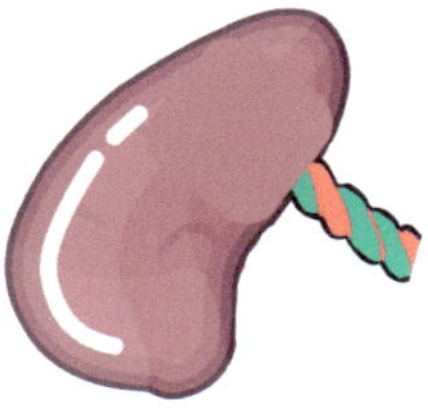

Lateral

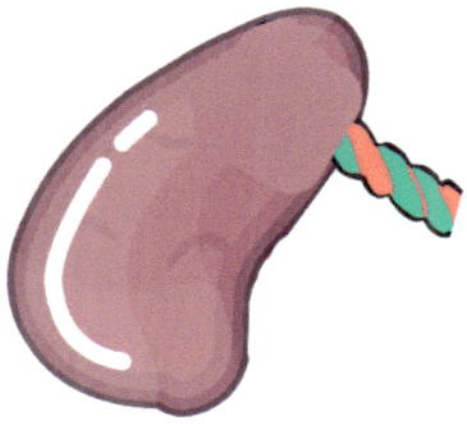

Marginal

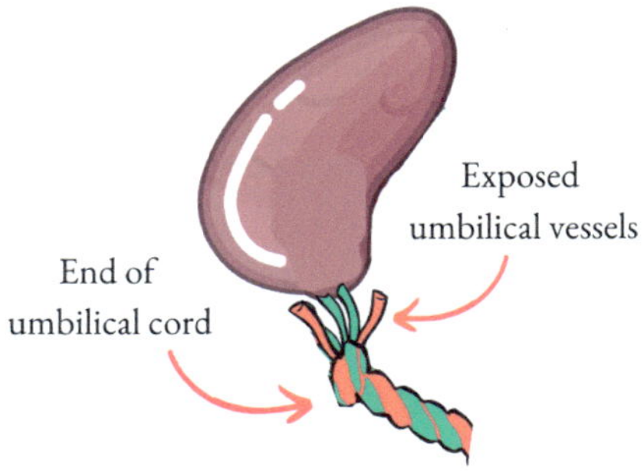

Velamentous

Notes

Notes

Notes

5

Pediatric Abdomen

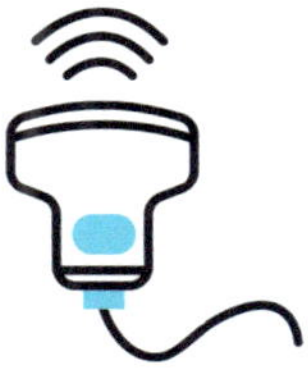

NEONATAL AND PEDIATRIC EXAMS can be challenging for many reasons. The patients may be crying, scared, guarded, combative, or maybe just move a lot. So don't be hard on yourself if it takes you a while to master them. Having a great mentor to help guide and teach you these exams is imperative, as they take a lot of practice and patience to master.

There is a lot to remember and the protocols can seem overwhelming. Bringing your mentor to shadow you until you feel comfortable doing these exams on your own is a great idea. When learning to do these exams, don't be scared to take cine clips so nothing is missed! It's ok to be extra cautious and very thorough.

Appendix

Patient Prep and Exam

No patient prep for this exam.

Transducers Used

- Linear ML6-15
- Linear 9L

Exam Indications

- RLQ px
- Nausea/vomiting
- Elevated WBC count
- Rebound Tenderness
- Fever

These are challenging exams because the appy (appendix) is hard to find. Don't be hard on yourself if it takes you a while to learn and accomplish this exam.

The appy location is different in everyone. Sometimes it sits over the right iliac artery and vein, sometimes it's more lateral to the bowel in the RLQ (right lower quadrant). In rarer occasions, it is located near the umbilicus or in the LLQ (left lower quadrant). Believe it or not, you can even find it near the kidney and liver!

Appendix

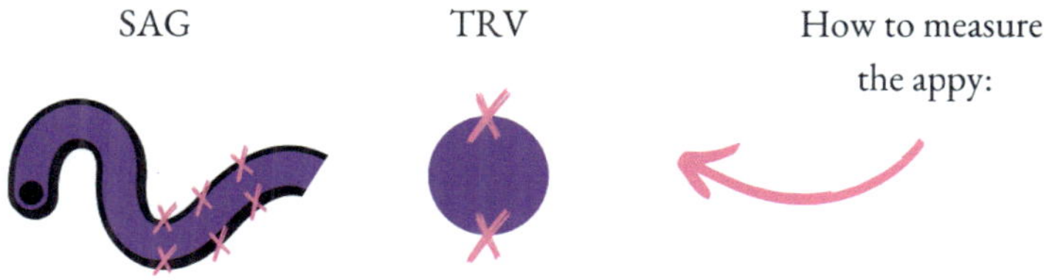

*Comes off the cecum

*Most common locations are
1. Adjacent to the right iliacs
2. In the RLQ lateral to the bowel

*Must find the BE (blind end)

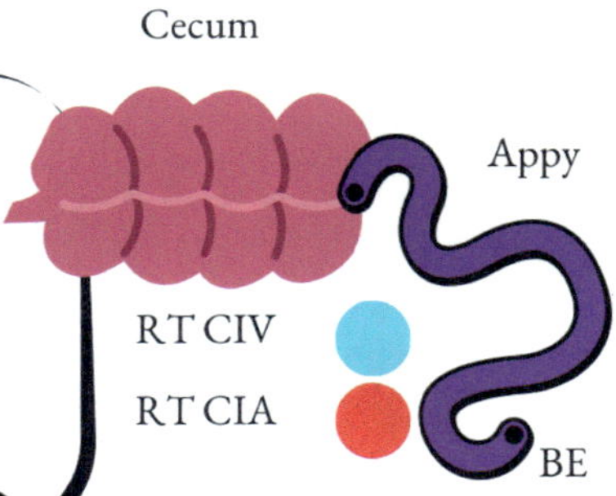

Abnormal Appendix:
AP: >6mm
Non-compressible
Hyperemic
FF in the RLQ or Morison's Pouch *Look at both locations!
LNs
Rebound Tenderness

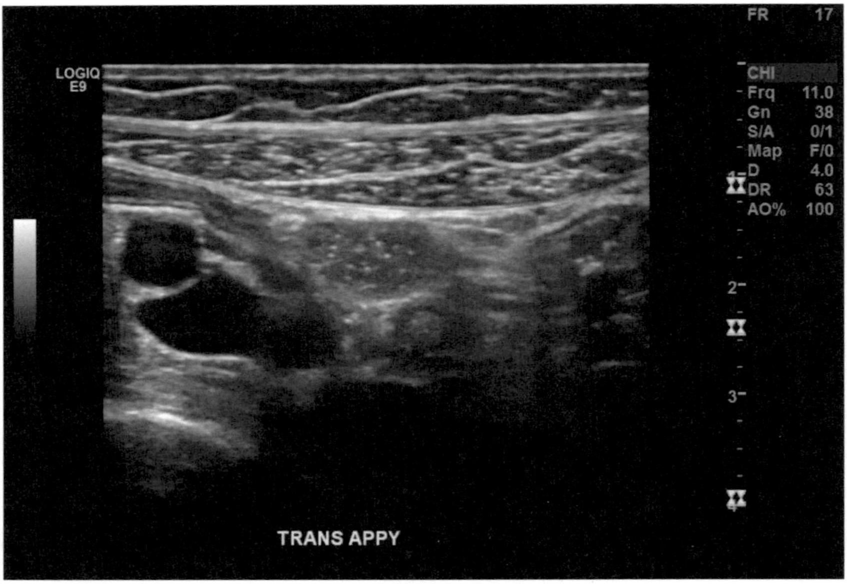

TRV appendix at the blind end

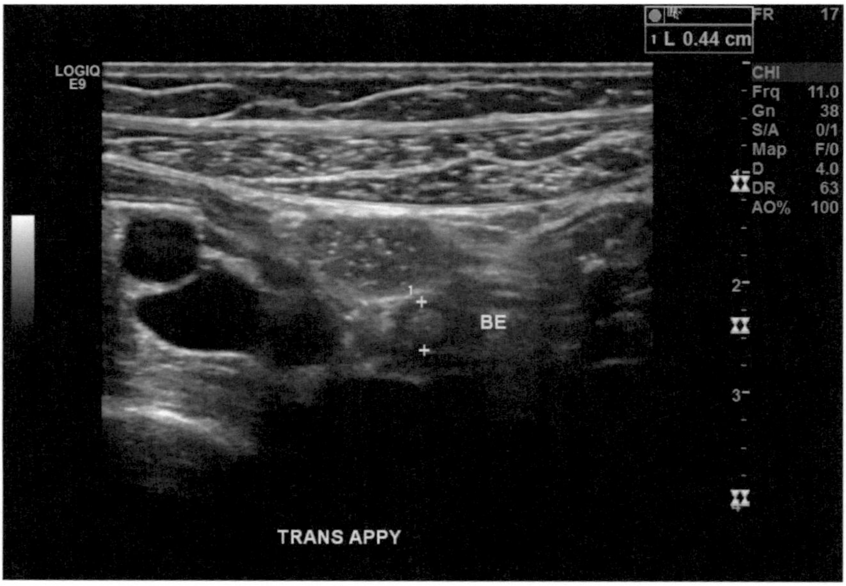

TRV appendix with AP measurement at the blind end

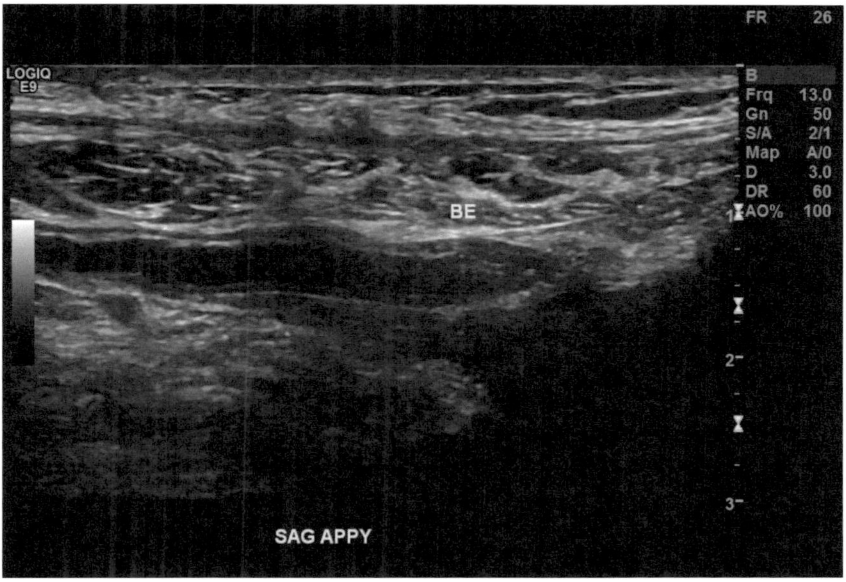

SAG appendix

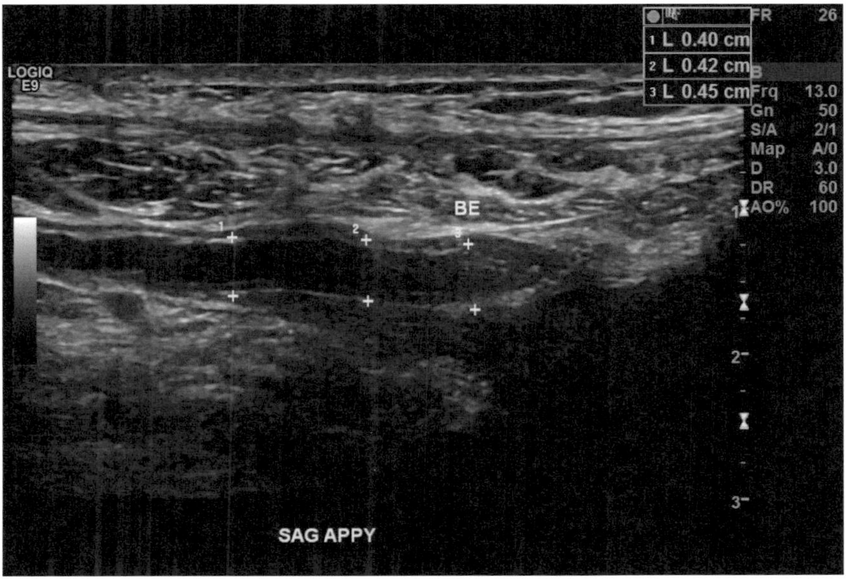

SAG appendix showing multiple measurements

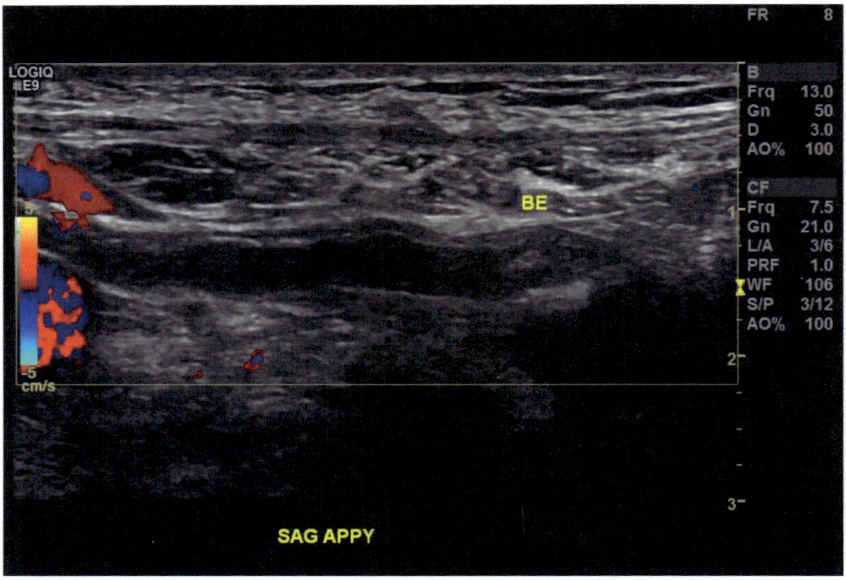

SAG appendix evaluated with color Doppler

Protocols

Appendix:

1. SAG Appy - coming off the cecum
   a. 2D
   b. Measurements: AP
   c. Color Doppler
   d. Cine clip
2. TRV Appy
   a. 2D (with and without compression. Include AP measurements)
   b. BE (blind end)
   c. Cine clip
3. Eval surrounding area for LNs and FF
   a. Measure the largest 3 LNs
   b. Document FF

I do a couple measurements along the SAG appy to find the largest segment

Intussusception

Patient Prep and Exam

The patient will need to by lying supine with their shirt lifted up or off to expose the abdomen.

Transducers Used

- Linear ML6-15

Exam Indications

- Intermittent abdominal px
- Vomiting
- Abdominal mass
- Bloody stool

Helpful Tips

Intussusception occurs when the intestines telescope in on themselves. In technical terms the intussusceptum is the prolapsed bowel that is pulled into the intussuscipiens (creating the "telescope"). The intussuscipiens is the bowel that receives the prolapsed bowel. The whole "telescope" is called intussusception and it presents as a "target sign".

There are two types of intussusception. The first kind, and most worrisome of the two, is ileocolic. The second is small bowel-small bowel. There are some differences between the two that help us determine which type of intussusception we are dealing with.

Ileocolic:

- Seen in the RLQ
- Larger in size
  - L: >3cm
  - AP: >2cm
- Will have a hyperechoic center (mesenteric fat gets pulled in)

Small bowel-small bowel:

- Seen elsewhere other than just the RLQ
- Smaller in size
  - L: < 3cm
  - AP: <2cm

It is important to evaluate the intestines for more than a few minutes, because intussusception can be intermittent and therefore might not be seen right away. When intussusception is observed measure both the length and AP diameter.

Intussusception

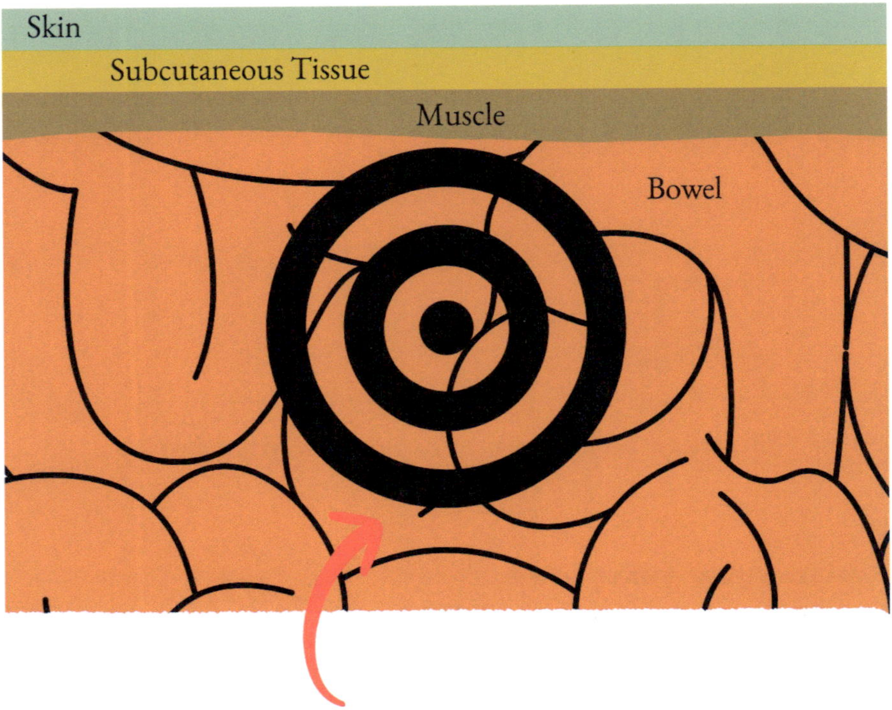

The telescoping effect of the intestines demonstrating the "Target Sign"

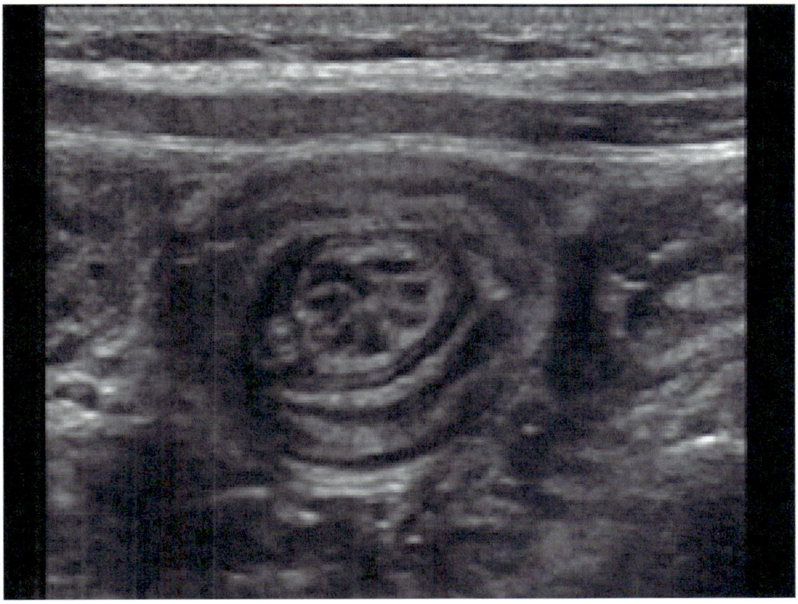

Intussusception. Image by UltrasoundCases.info and SonoSkills.com

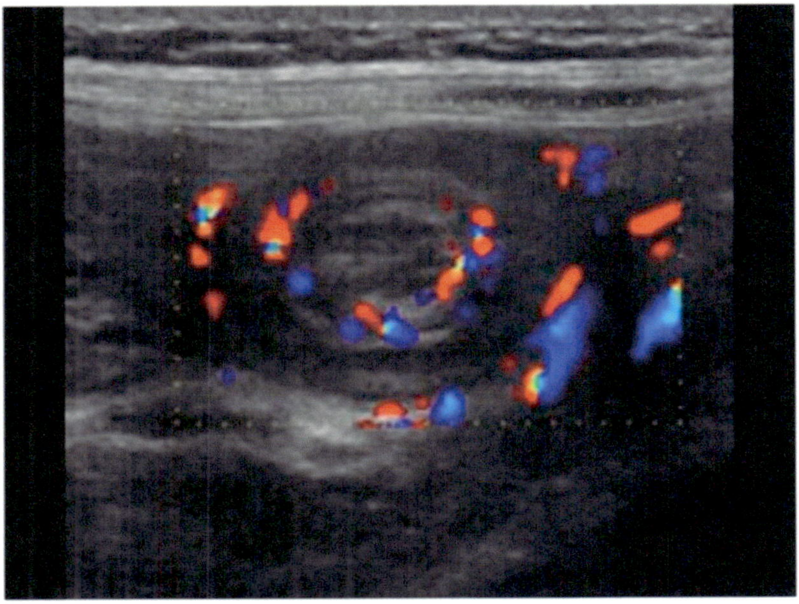

Intussusception evaluated with color Doppler. Image by UltrasoundCases.info and SonoSkills.com

Protocols

Intussusception:

1. RUQ
2. LUQ
3. LLQ
4. RLQ
5. ML
   a. Sup
   b. Mid
   c. Inf

In each of the 4 quadrants, you will take SAG and TRV images. You will take TRV images midline at sup, mid, and inf

If intussusception is seen, measure the L + AP and evaluate with color Doppler

Pyloric Stenosis

Patient Prep and Exam

The patient needs to be NPO for about 4 hours. Bowel gas is the enemy during this exam.

Transducers Used

- Linear ML6-15
- Linear 9L

Exam Indications

- Projectile vomiting
- Palpable lump
- Weight loss

Helpful Tips

Gas can be an issue when scanning the pylorus. To help get around it, you can gently increase the transducer pressure to squish the bowel away or you can RLD the patient to help move the gas away. This exam is quite challenging when babies are fussy, so they do tend to take a little bit of time.

Normal Measurements

Structure:	Abbreviation/Acronym:	Measurements:
Pylorus	-	**Muscle Wall:** AP: <3mm **TRV Pylorus:** AP: <14mm **Pyloric Channel:** L: <15mm

Pyloric Stenosis

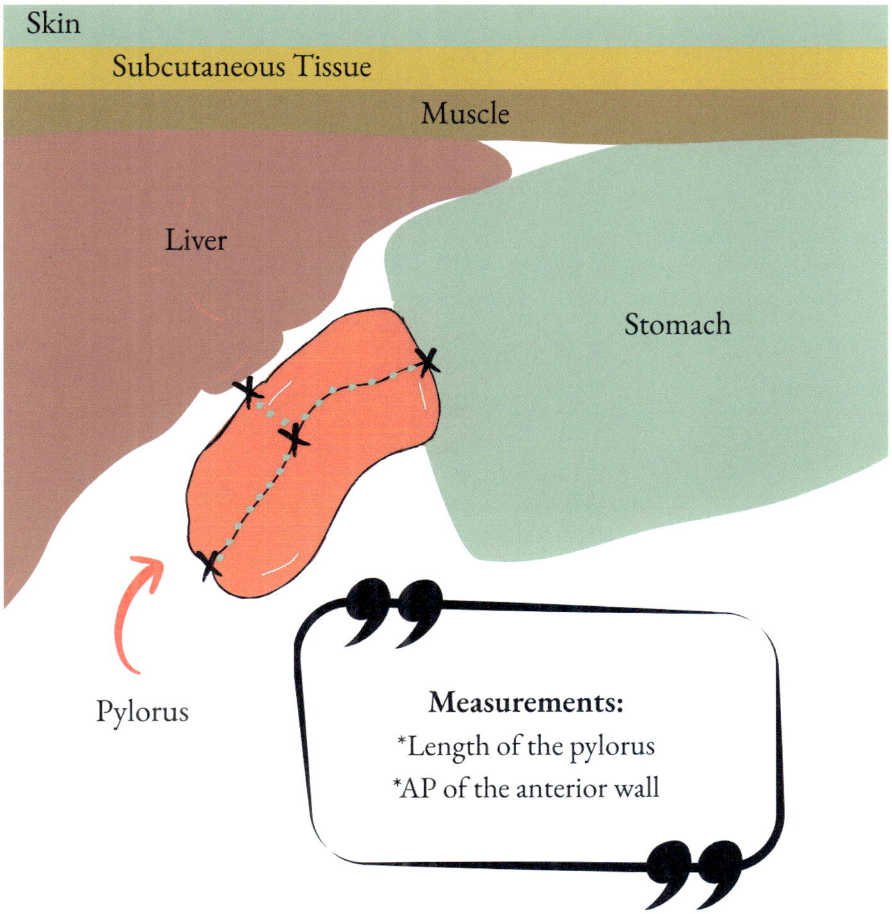

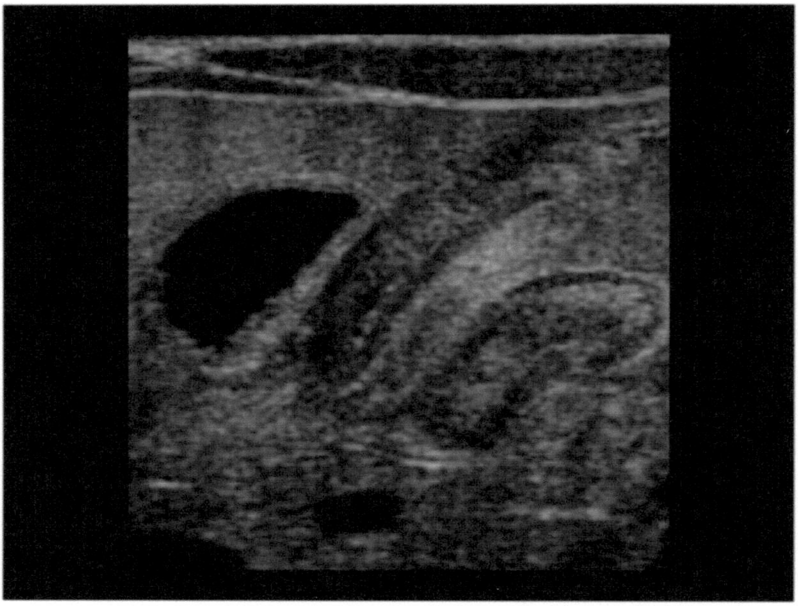

Pyloric stenosis in SAG. Image by UltrasoundCases.info and SonoSkills.com

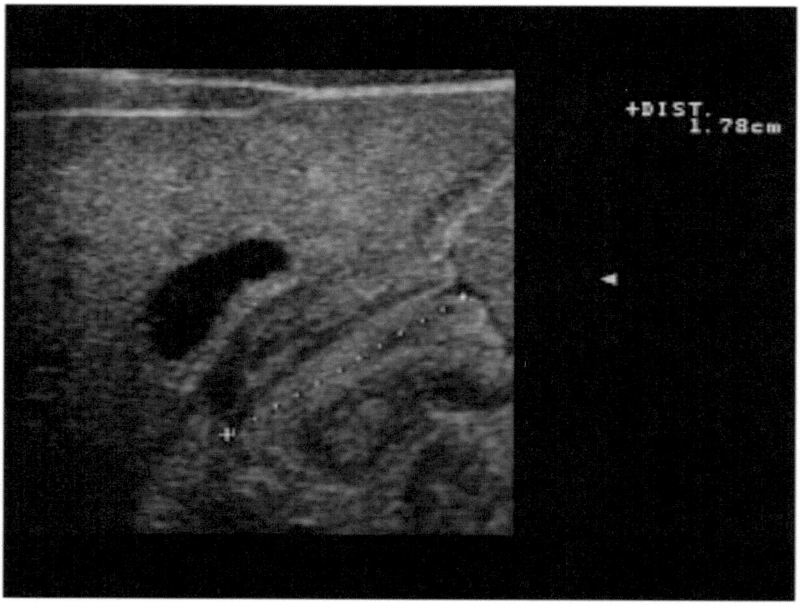

Pyloric stenosis in SAG with measurement. Image by UltrasoundCases.info and SonoSkills.com

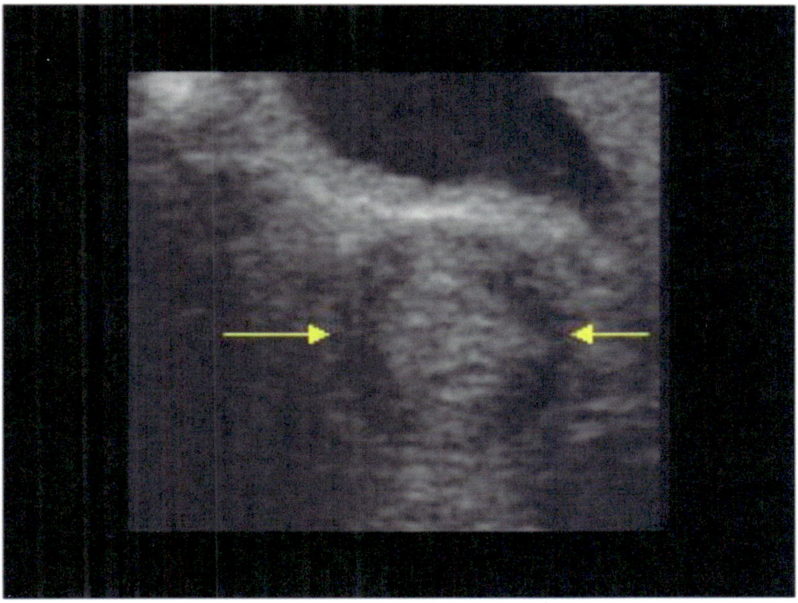

Pyloric stenosis in TRV. Image by UltrasoundCases.info and SonoSkills.com

Protocols

Pyloric Stenosis:

1. TRV Pylorus
    a. 2D
    b. Measurements:
        i. Pylorus: AP
2. SAG Pylorus
    a. 2D
    b. Measurements: L + AP anterior wall
3. SAG Pylorus
    a. Cine clip evaluating food passing through the pylorus and into the duodenum

Between steps 2 and 3 you will feed the baby. There is a special food for this and will be located in your department

Pediatric Abdomen + Pelvis + Small Parts

Patient Prep and Exam

Abdomen

The patient needs to be NPO for 6+ hours.

Pelvis

The patient needs to arrive with a full bladder.

Small Parts

The area of concern needs to be accessible. If it is a head and neck or chest/back, the shirt may need to come off or lifted up. If the exam is for a scrotum, then the pants and underwear/diaper need to be removed.

Transducers Used

Abdomen

- Linear ML6-15
- Curvilinear C1-6
- Linear L8-18i (Hockey stick)

Pelvis

- Linear ML6-15
- Curvilinear C1-6

Small Parts

- Linear ML6-15

Exam Indications

Abdomen

- Px
- Lump
- Nausea/vomiting

Pelvis

- Px
- Palpable mass

Small Parts

- Undescended testicles
- Px
- Palpable thyroid
- Palpable lump
- Swelling

Protocols

Protocols are the same for pediatrics as they are for adults. Refer to each of the following chapters below to find the protocols.

Abdomen

See Chapter 1: Abdomen for protocols.

Pelvis

See Chapter 6: Pelvis – GYN for protocols.

Small Parts

See Chapter 7: Small Parts for protocols.

Notes

Notes

Notes

6

Pelvis - GYN

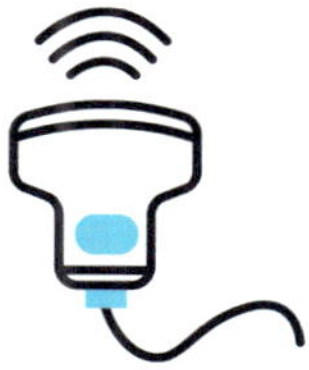

Patient Prep and Exam

This exam is done transabdominally (TA) and transvaginally (TV). TA is done on top of the pelvis with the curvilinear transducer, where the TV is done with the transvaginal transducer.

The patient needs to come to the exam with a full bladder. The full bladder is used as a window for the TA portion of the exam. After the TA, the patient will empty their bladder for the TV portion of the exam. Having a full bladder during the TV exam is a pitfall, as it makes imaging much more difficult and lower quality. A full bladder will actually push the organs out of view.

Transducers Used

- Curvilinear C1-6
- Transvaginal Transducer IC5-9

Exam Indications

- Px
- Lump
- VB (vaginal bleeding)
- AUB (abnormal uterine bleeding)
- PMB (post-menopausal bleeding)
- IUD check

Functions and Labs

<table>
<tr><th>Structure:</th><th>Function:</th><th>Labs:</th></tr>
<tr><td>Endometrium</td><td>Is the inner most lining of the uterus

Area of ovum implantation

If fertilization does not occur, the endo is shed during menses</td><td rowspan="3">Estrogen
Progesterone
hCG: <25 = not pregnant
WBC</td></tr>
<tr><td>Ovaries</td><td>Produces estrogen and progesterone

Produces eggs for fertilization</td></tr>
<tr><td>Uterus</td><td>If fertilization occurs, it provides the location for the fetus to grow

If fertilization does not occur, then the uterus will shed the endometrium, then prepare for the next cycle</td></tr>
</table>

Hot Topic Question: Who Do We TV!?

Let's briefly discuss who we TV, since this is a hot topic question and conversation. Listen... everyone you ask will have a different answer to this question. Instead of giving you my own personal thoughts on it, I will just tell you how my department runs.

Every single person who comes in for a transvaginal ultrasound will need to sign a consent form when checking in. We then grab the patient, go over the consent form, and I personally, get verbal consent as well in the US room. I then must sign and date the consent form prior to doing the transvaginal US. If the patient does NOT sign the consent form, we do NOT perform the TV US.

Let's say the patient is over 18 (NOT A MINOR) but is not sexually active. We still give the consent form to the patient. We discuss the exam and leave it up to the patient if they would like to proceed with the transvaginal exam. If the patient consents to the exam, we do it. If the patient does not, then obviously we do not do the exam.

Let's say the patient is under 18 (IS A MINOR) and not sexually active, we do NOT perform the TV US. If the patient is under 18 (IS A MINOR) and is sexually active, then we must have consent from both the patient and a parent or guardian and they both must sign the consent form.

This is the first facility that I have worked for that has a consent form for the TV exam. However, I think it is a great idea. I feel that at some point in the future, this will become standard practice.

Uterine Positions

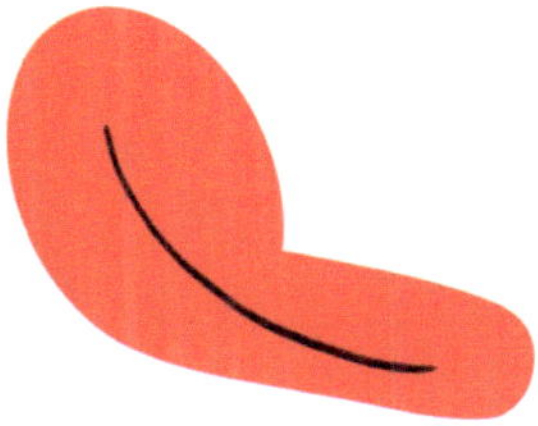

Anteverted

Fundus faces up

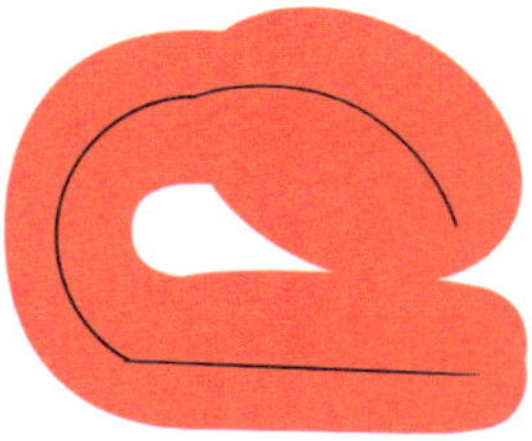

Anteflexed

Fundus faces up and touches the cx

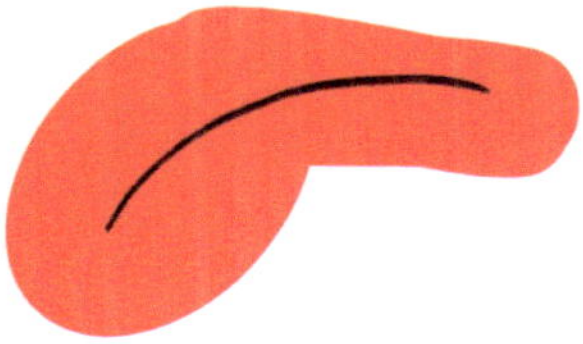

Retroverted

Fundus faces down

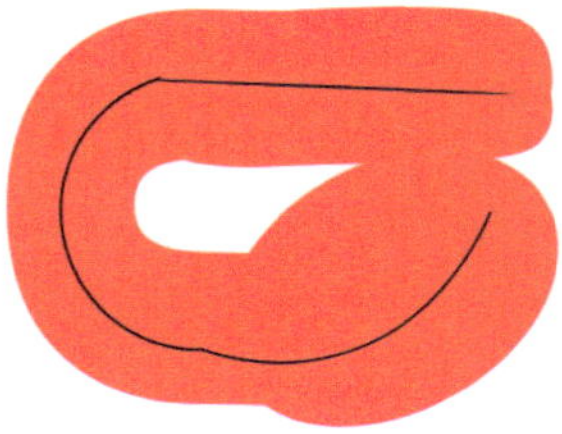

Retroflexed

Fundus faces down and touches the cx

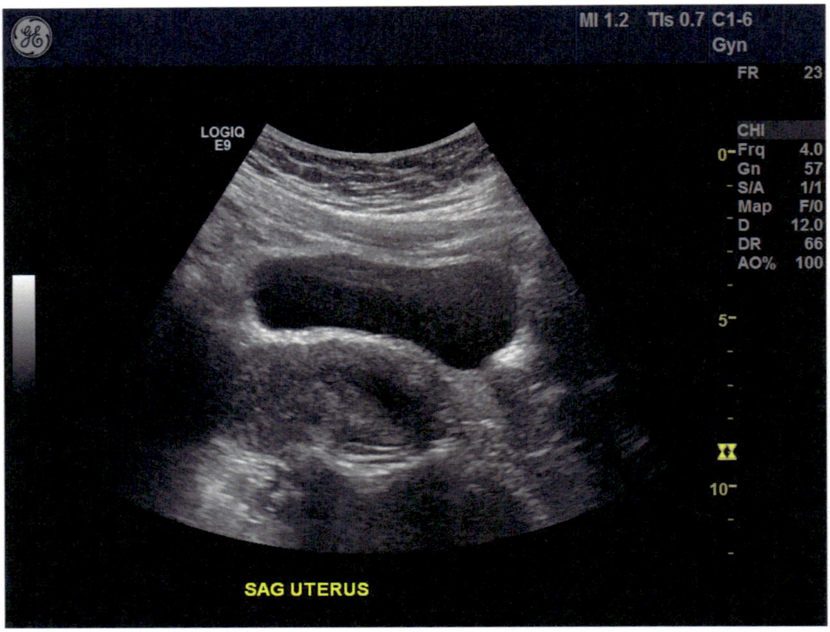

Transabdominal view of a retroverted uterus

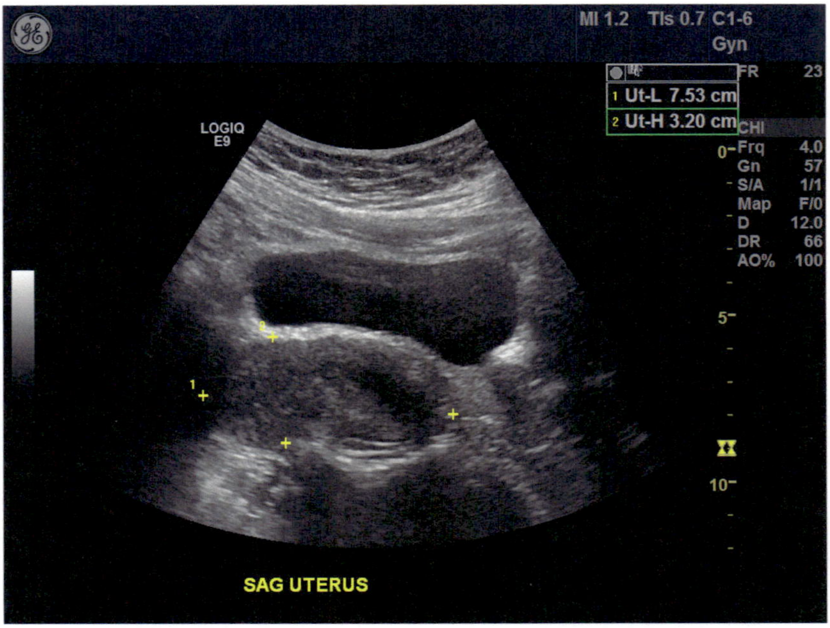

Transabdominal view of a retroverted uterus with measurements

Normal Measurements

Structure:	Abbreviation/Acronym:	Measurements:
Cervix	CX	2-4cm
Endometrium	ENDO	
Menstrual Phases: • Menstruation (days 1-5) • Early Proliferative (days 6-10) • Late proliferative (days 11-14) • Secretory (days 15-28)		• Menstruation: 2-4mm • Early prolif: 5-7mm • Late prolif: »11mm • Secretory: 7-16mm
Post-menopause	POST-MENO	<5mm
Hormone Replacement Therapy	HRT	<8mm
Post Dilation and Curettage or Abortion	D&C or AB	<5mm
Ovaries	RO or LO	
Follicles		<2.5cm
Menstrual Cycle	MENSES	L: <3cm AP: <2cm W: <3cm Vol: »9.8ml
Post-menopause	POST-MENO	L: <2cm Vol: »2.8ml

Normal Measurements Continued

Structure:	Abbreviation/Acronym:	Measurements:
Uterus	UT	
Nulliparous		L: 6-8cm H: 3-5cm W: 3-5cm
Parous		L: 8-10cm H: 5-6cm W: 5-6cm
Post-menopause	POST-MENO	L: 3-5cm H: 2-3cm W: 2-3cm

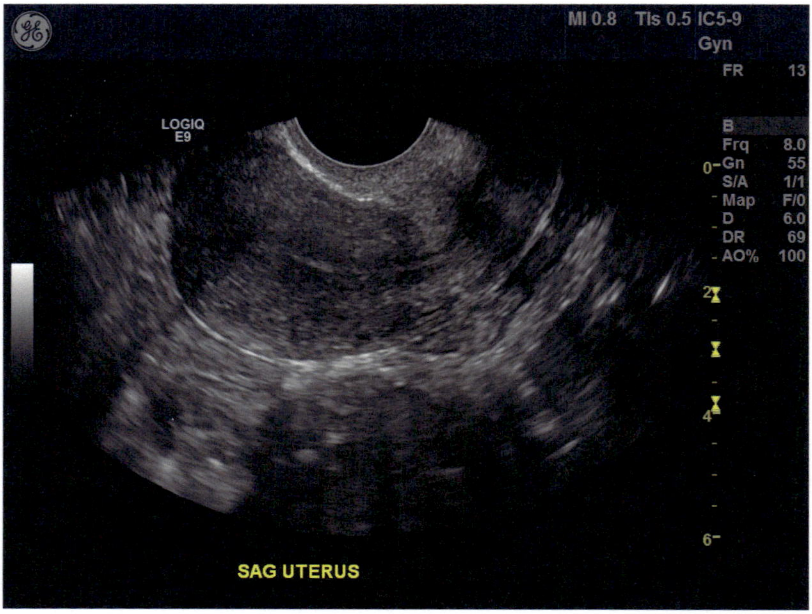

Transvaginal view of an anteverted uterus

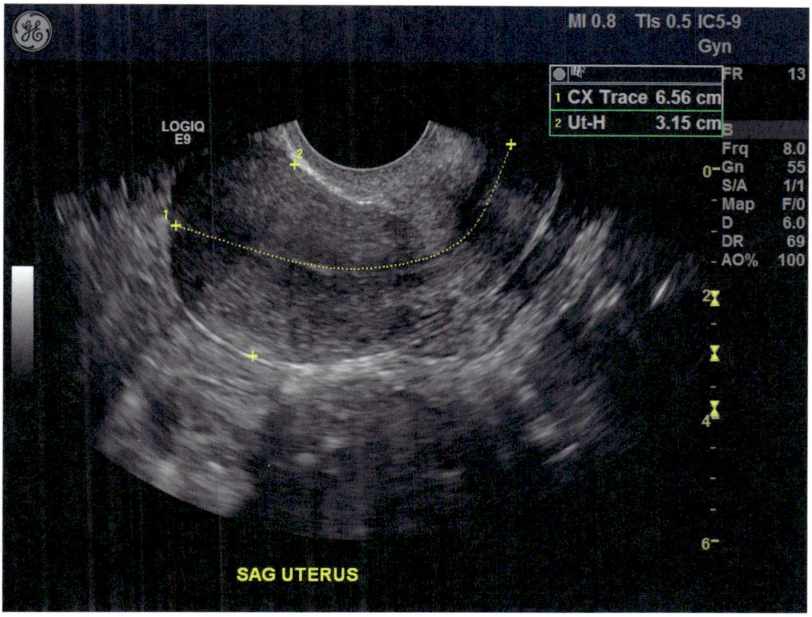

Transvaginal view of an anteverted uterus with measurements

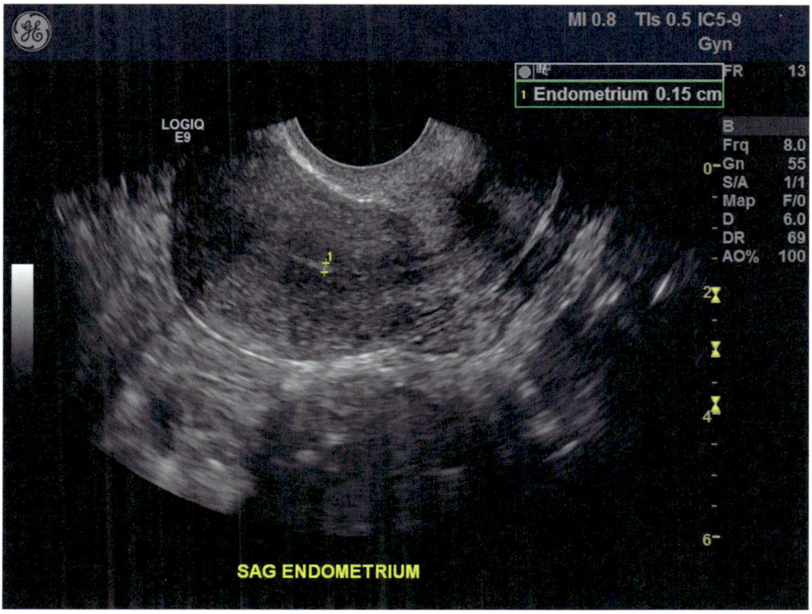

Transvaginal view of a SAG endometrium with measurement

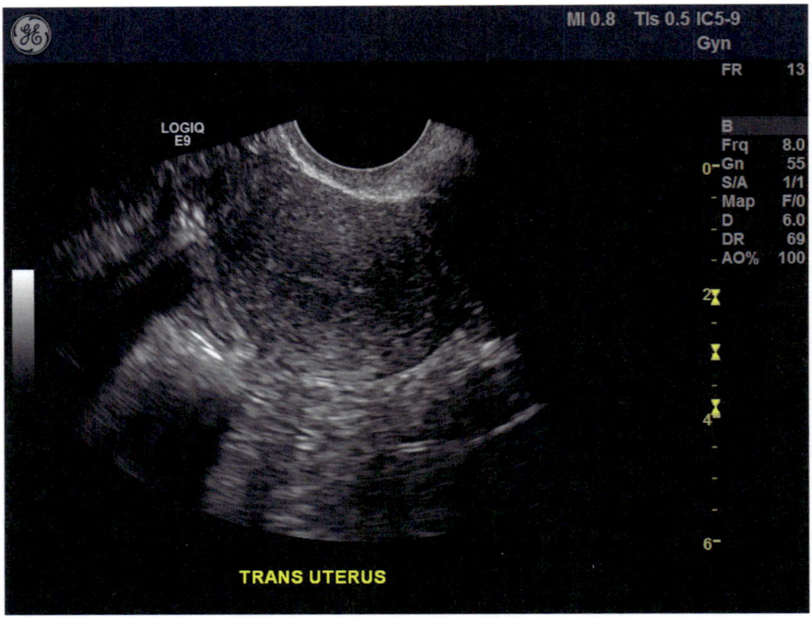

Transvaginal view of a TRV uterus

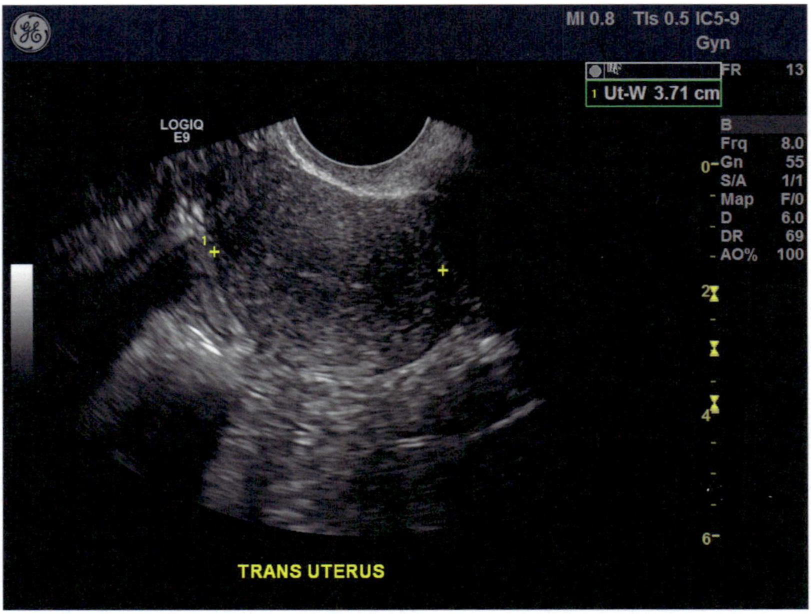

Transvaginal view of a TRV uterus with measurement

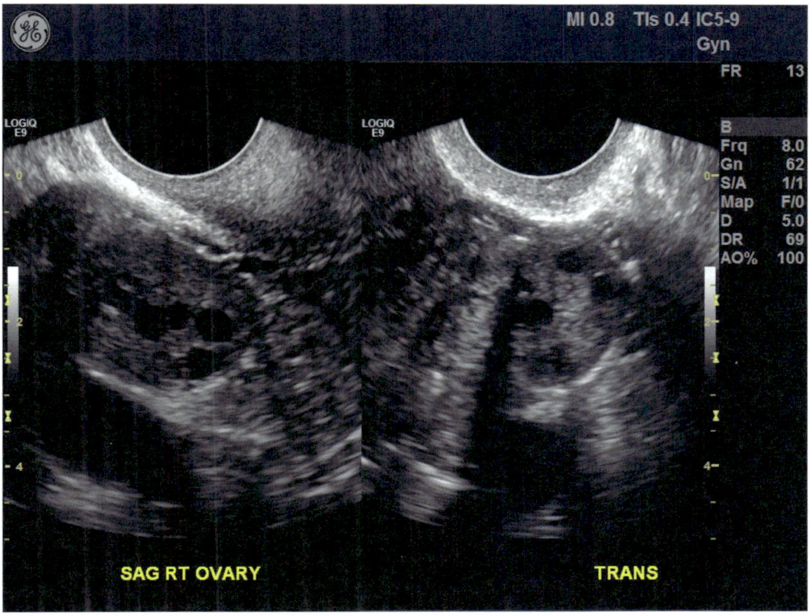

Transvaginal view of the SAG + TRV right ovary

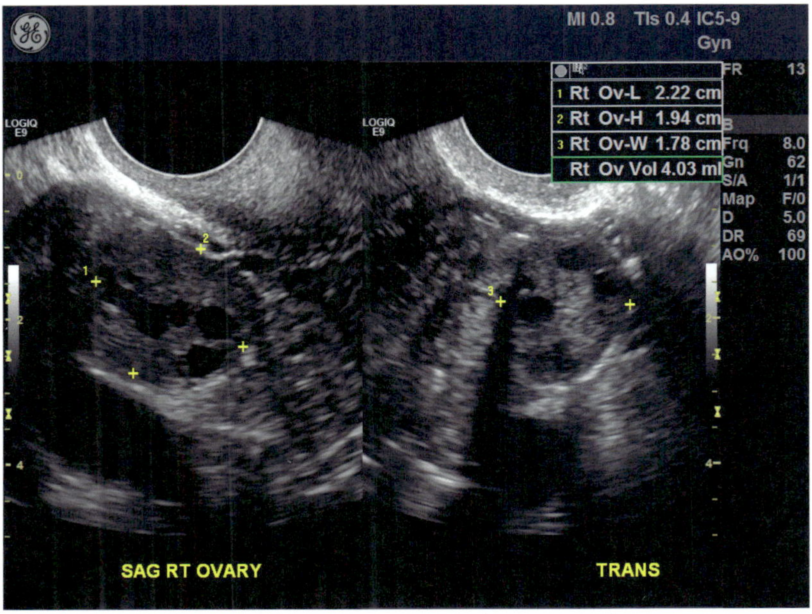

Transvaginal view of the SAG + TRV right ovary with measurements

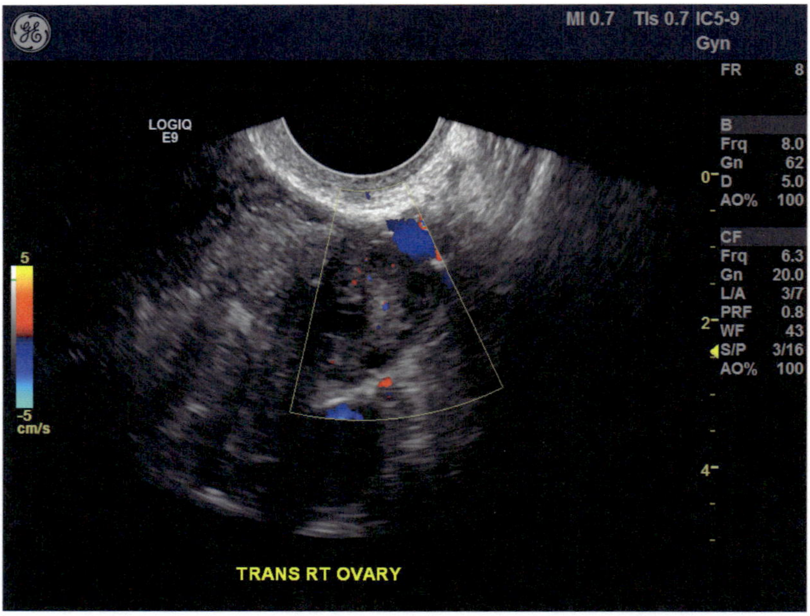

Transvaginal view of the right ovary evaluated with color Doppler

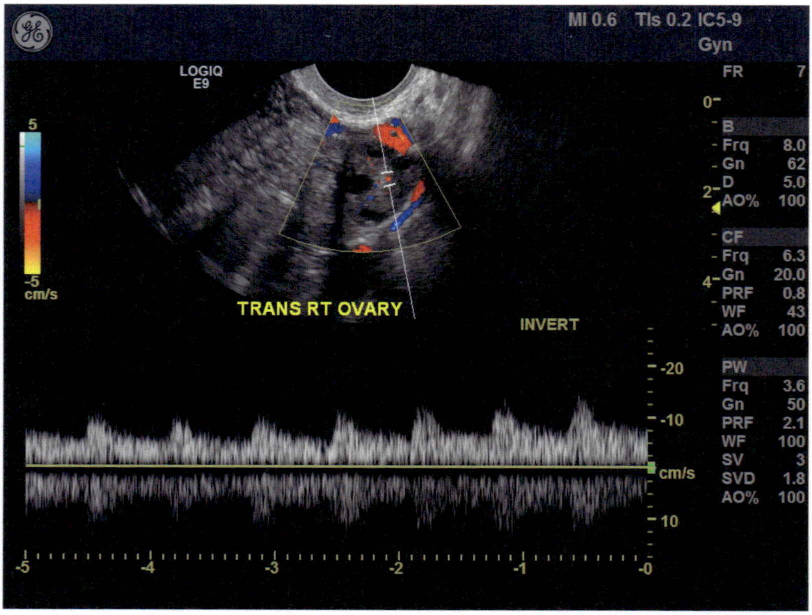

Transvaginal view of the right ovary evaluated with color and spectral Doppler

Protocols

Pelvis with Transvaginal:

Both the TA and TV exams have the exact same protocol. Start with the TA exam first, then once done, do the TV exam

If the patient has an IUD, make sure to document that in both TA and TV exams

1. SAG UT
    a. 2D
    b. Measurements: L + AP
    c. 2D: RT - LT
2. SAG ENDO
    a. 2D
    b. Measurements: AP
    c. Color Doppler
3. SAG CX
4. TRV CX
5. TRV UT
    a. 2D: Inf - Sup
    b. Measurements: W
6. SAG / TRV RT O
    a. 2D
    b. Measurements: L + AP + W
    c. Color Doppler
    d. Spectral Doppler
7. SAG / TRV LT O
    a. 2D
    b. Measurements: L + AP + W
    c. Color Doppler
    d. Spectral Doppler
8. SAG CDS

Some places evaluate ovarian blood flow with spectral Doppler as their normal protocol, not just to rule out torsion

Notes

Notes

Notes

7

Small Parts

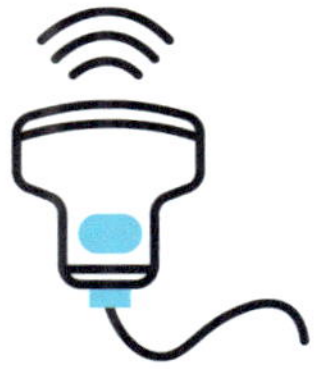

Head and Neck

Patient Prep and Exam

No patient prep.

Transducers Used

- Linear ML6-15

Exam Indications

- Palpable lump / swelling
- Px

Functions

<table>
<tr><th>Structure:</th><th>Function:</th></tr>
<tr><td>Lymph Node</td><td>Part of the immune system

Transfers lymph throughout the body through the lymphatic system</td></tr>
<tr><td>Parotid</td><td rowspan="2">Produces saliva

Helps aid digestion, helps with swallowing, and helps protect teeth from bacteria</td></tr>
<tr><td>Submandibular</td></tr>
</table>

Helpful Tips

Some things to note about lymph nodes is that they're considered "normal" vs "abnormal" using the short-axis measurement rather than the length measurement. For lymph nodes NOT in the submandibular and inguinal region, that normal measurement is <1cm. For lymph nodes IN the submandibular and inguinal region, they can be up to 1.5cm in the short axis.

Another thing to note, is that lymph node morphology is more important when determining if they are normal vs abnormal than actual size. So what constitutes a normal lymph node?

<u>Normal Lymph Node:</u>

- Thin cortex: <3mm
- Fatty hilum

- Oval / kidney shaped
- Hilar blood flow

Abnormal Lymph Node:

- Thick cortex: >3mm
- Lobular/irregular cortex
- Heterogenous
- Loss of fatty hilum
- Round
- Hyperemic

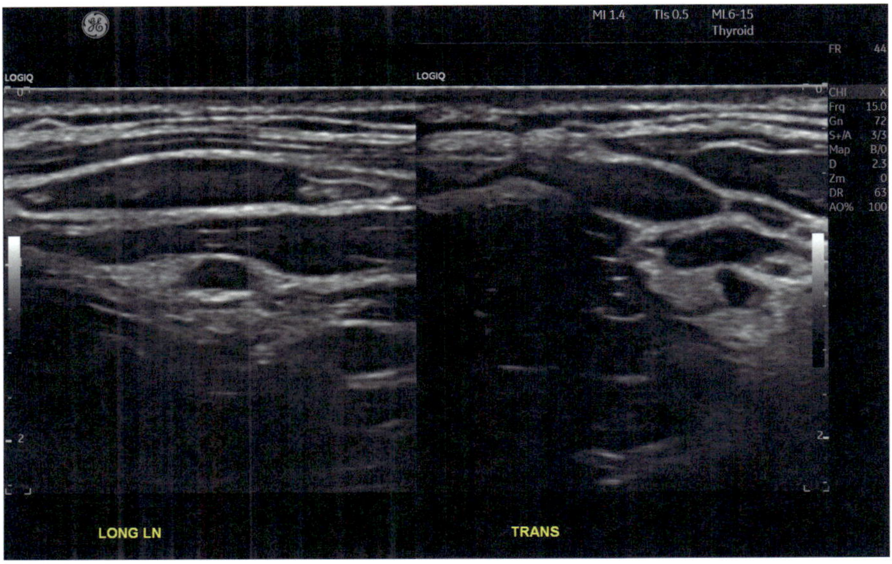

SAG + TRV lymph node

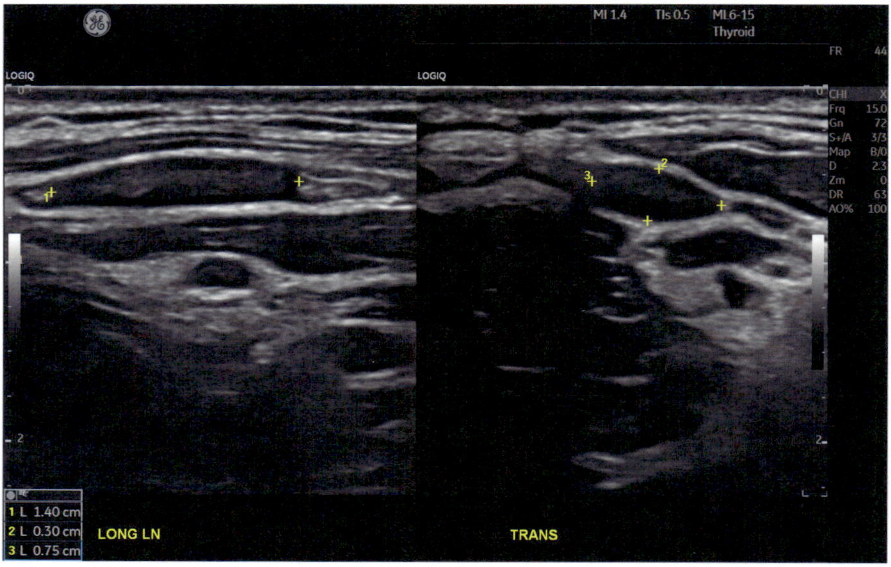

SAG + TRV lymph node with measurements

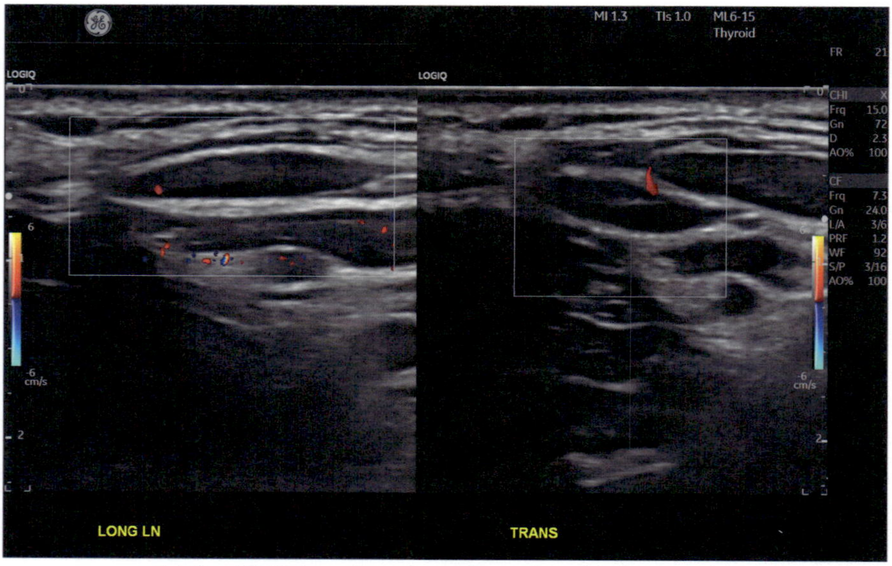

SAG + TRV lymph node evaluated with color Doppler

Normal Measurements

Structure:	Abbreviation/Acronym:	Measurements:
Lymph Node	LN	L: <2cm W: <1cm Submand + Inguinal Region: W: <1.5cm Cortex: <3mm
Parotid		4.6 x 3.7 x 2.2cm Vol: 19.6ml
Submandibular	SUBMAND	3.3 x 1.4 x 3.5cm Vol: 8.5ml

Salivary Glands

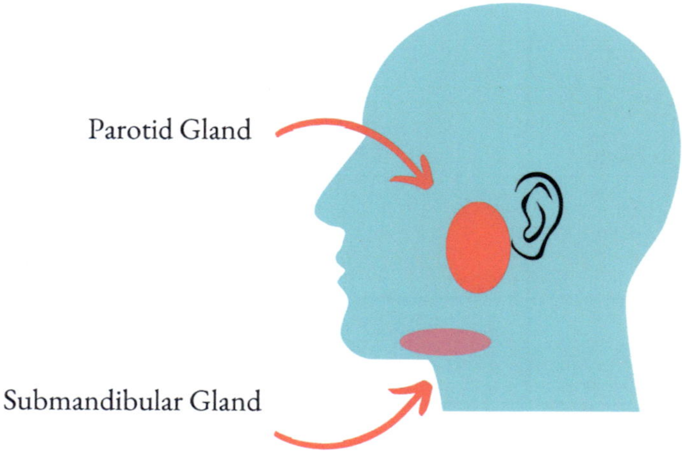

Lymph Node

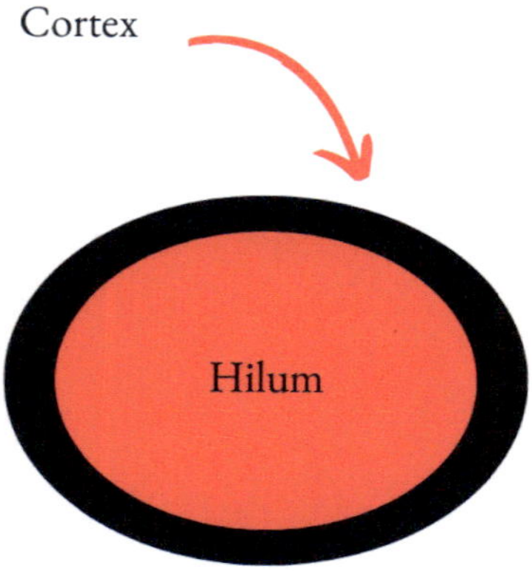

Thyroid Gland

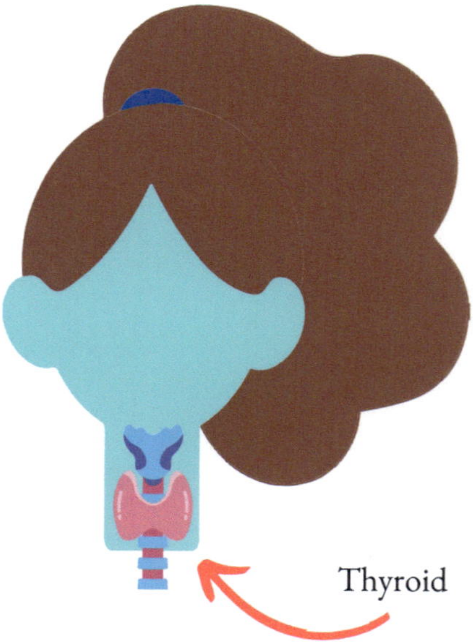

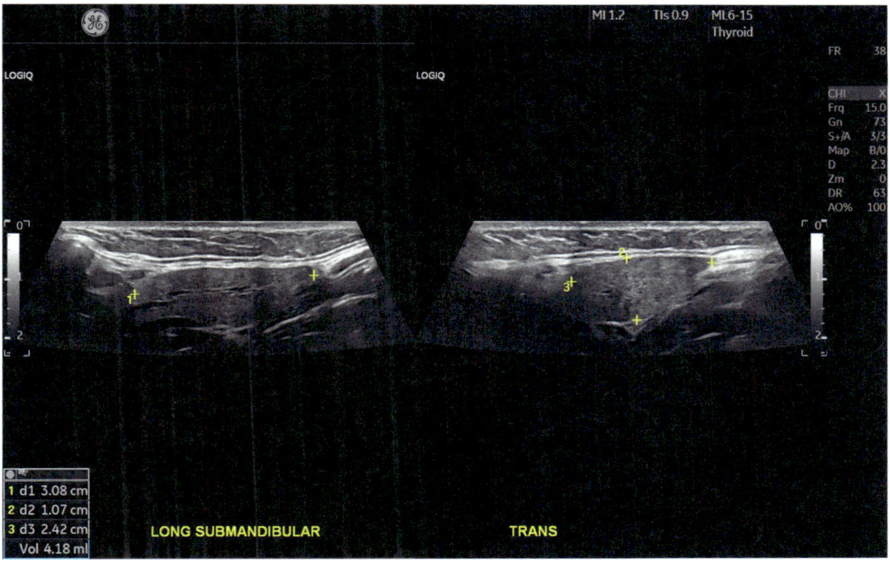

SAG + TRV submandibular gland with measurements

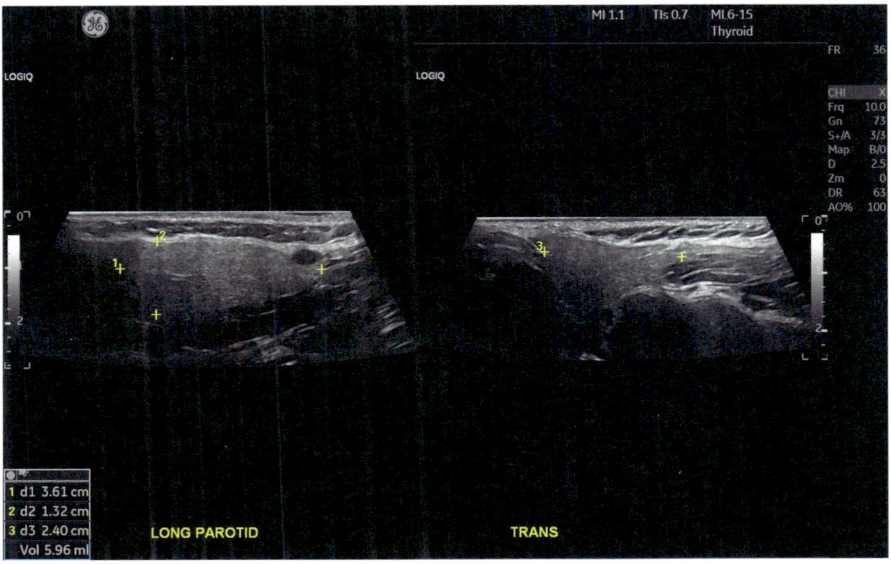

SAG + TRV parotid gland with measurements

Protocols

Lymph Nodes:

1. 2D
2. Measurements: L + AP + W
3. Color Doppler (demonstrate hilar blood flow)

These images will be done in dual-screen with SAG on the left and TRV on the right

Salivary Glands:

1. 2D
2. Measurements: L + AP + W (calculate a volume)
3. Color Doppler
4. Evaluate for abnormal LNs
   a. 2D
   b. Measurements: L + AP + W
   c. Color Doppler

The parotid and submandibular salivary glands are evaluated the same way, obtaining the same images. These images will be done in dual-screen with SAG on the left and TRV on the right

Scrotum

Patient Prep and Exam

No patient prep.

Transducers Used

- Linear ML6-15

Exam Indications

- Px
- Swelling
- Lump
- Infection
- Skin discoloration

Functions and Labs

Structure:	Function:	Labs:
Epididymis	Stores and transports sperm from the testicles	WBC
Testicle	Produces sperm Produces testosterone	WBC
Prostate	Secretes an alkaline fluid that is combined with sperm to help neutralize the acidity of the vagina, uterus, and fallopian tubes	PSA

Helpful Tips

There is no right or wrong way to set up the patient for this exam. Some sonographers use the "hammock" method, where the scrotum rests on a towel that is then tucked around the patient's waist. This suspends the scrotum between the thighs, rather than being stuck low and unable to reach. Some have the patient cross their legs with their scrotum resting on top of the thighs. Some have the patient do nothing and just scan them in whatever position the patient is most comfortable in. Do what works best for you!

Quick Tip! Have the patient lay as close to you on the stretcher as possible. This keeps you from reaching and causing strain on your neck, shoulder, and back.

Keep in mind that we need to keep the patient as covered as possible. The best way to do this is to have the patient cover their penis with a towel, and you can lay a towel, gown, blanket, or sheet over their legs. I found this to be a great way to make them feel more comfortable and not so exposed during the exam.

Normal Measurements

Structure:	Abbreviation/Acronym:	Measurements:
Epididymis	EPI	L: 3.8cm Head: 0.6-1.5cm *Typically, only the head is measured
Testicle	TEST	L: 3-5cm AP: 2-3cm W: 2-4cm
Prostate	PROST	L: 4cm AP: 3cm W:4cm Vol: 25ml

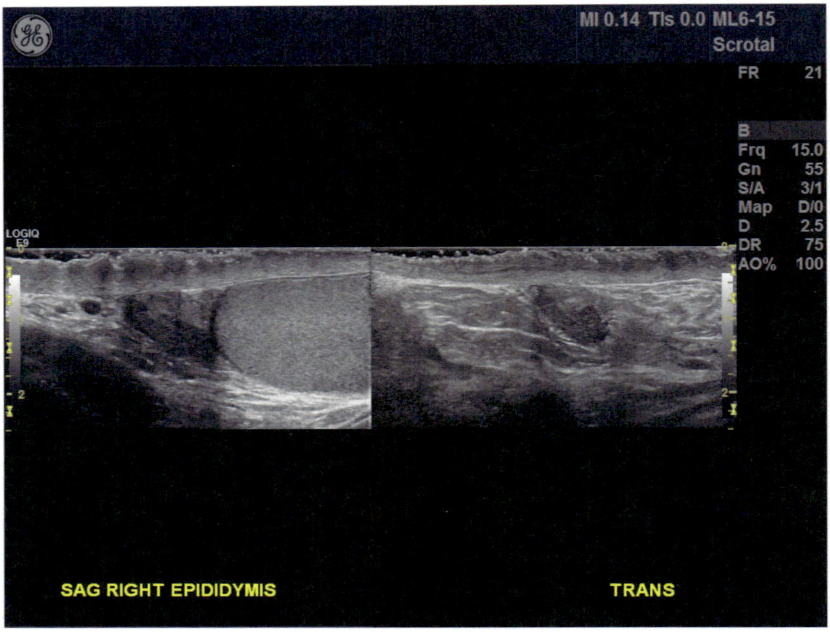

SAG + TRV right epididymis

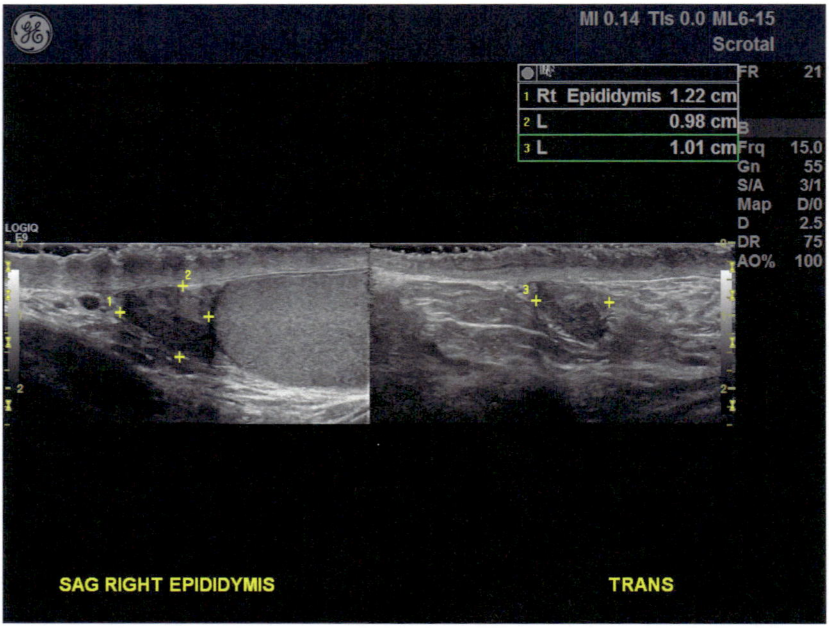

SAG + TRV right epididymis with measurements

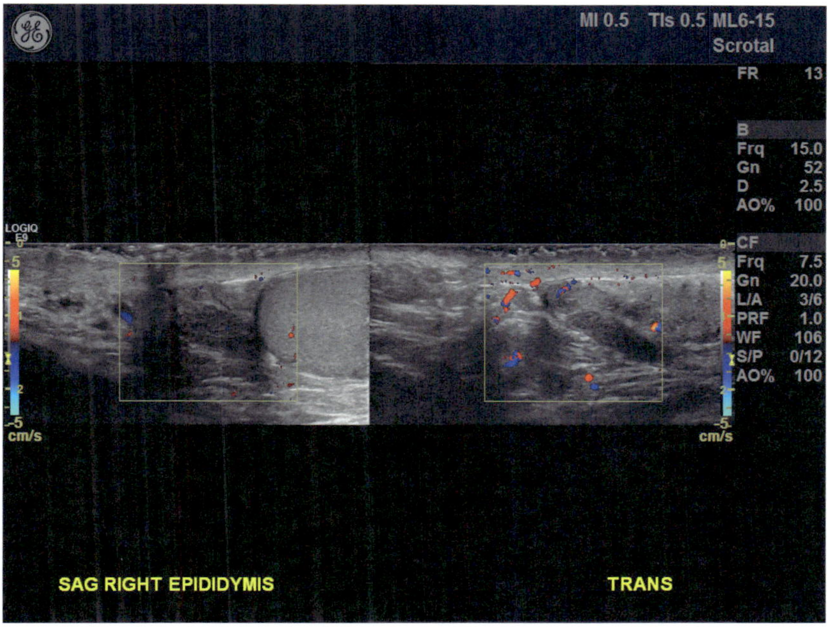

SAG + TRV right epididymis evaluated with color Doppler

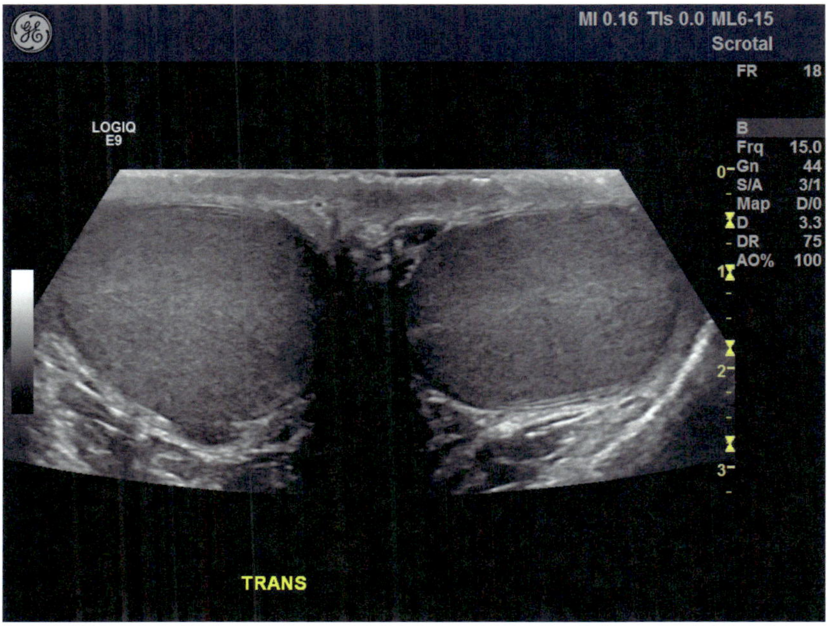

Bilateral testicle "Buddy" image

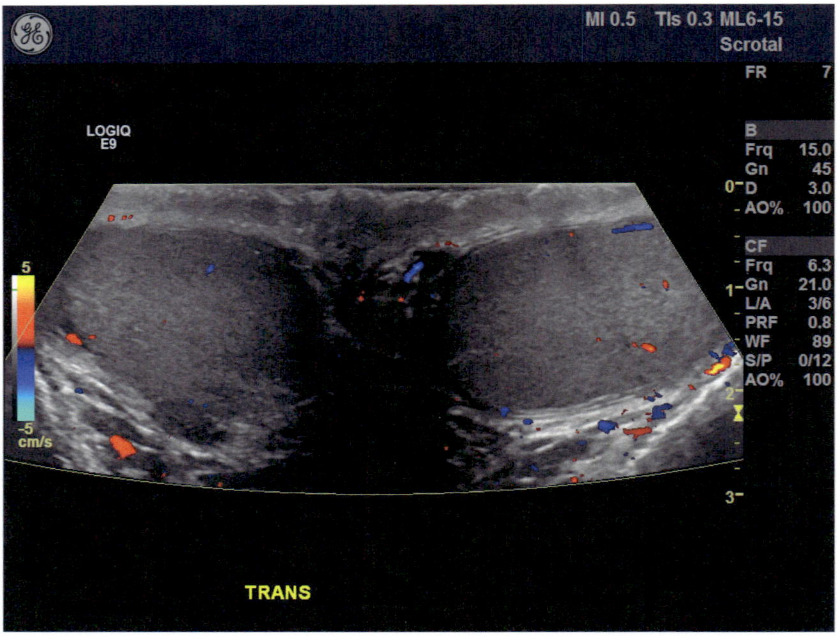

Bilateral testicle "Buddy" image evaluated with color Doppler

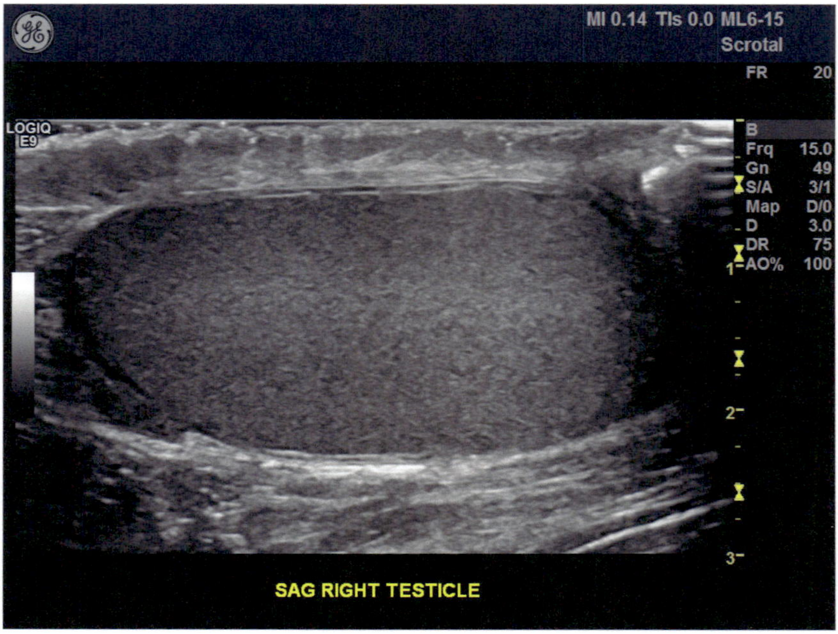

SAG right testicle

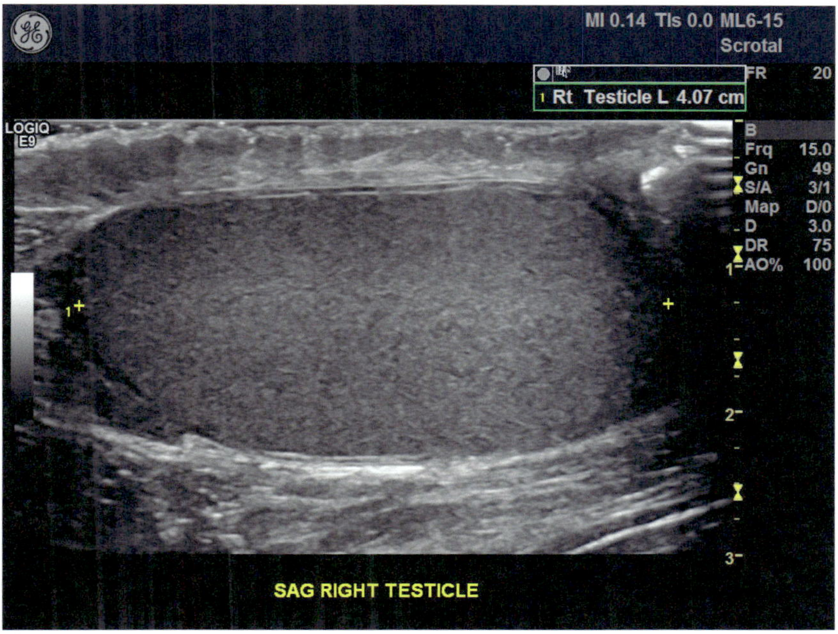

SAG right testicle with measurement

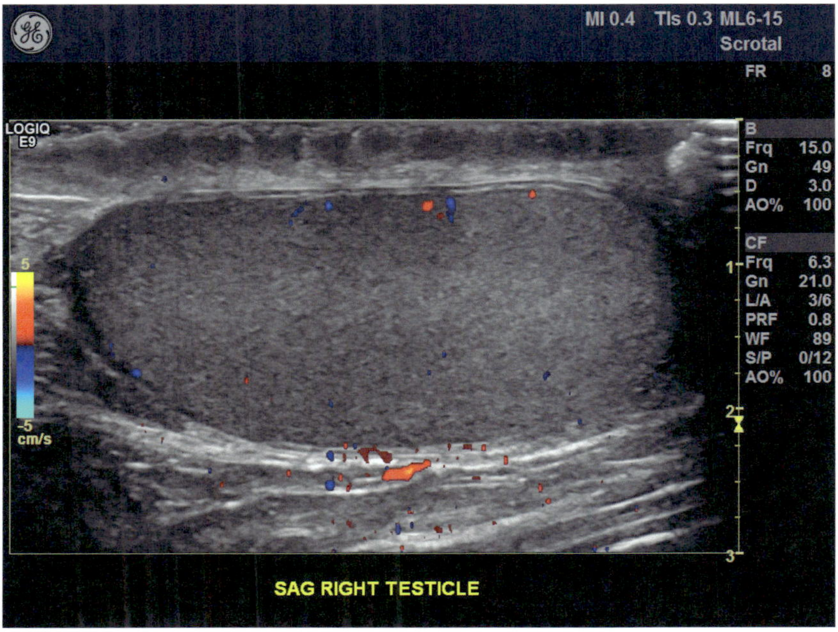

SAG right testicle evaluated with color Doppler

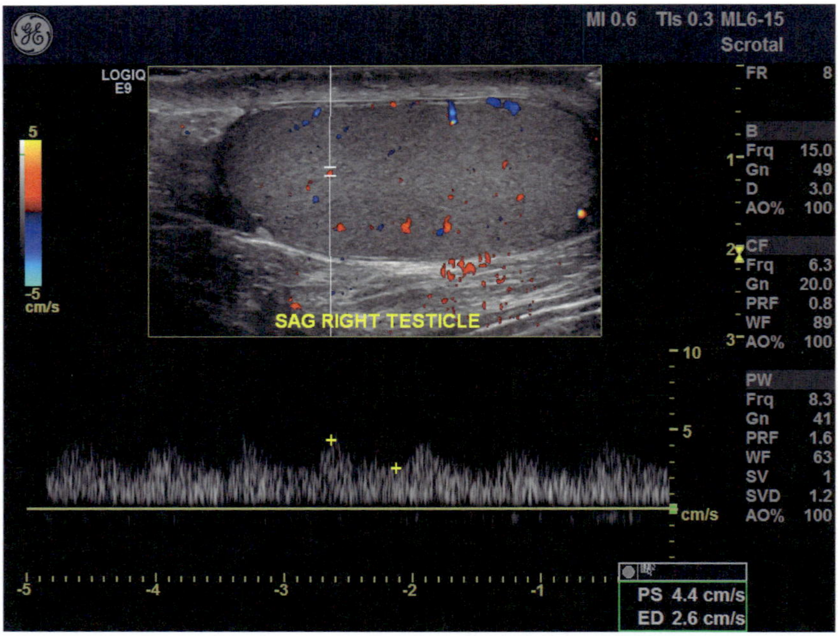

SAG right testicle evaluated with color and spectral Doppler

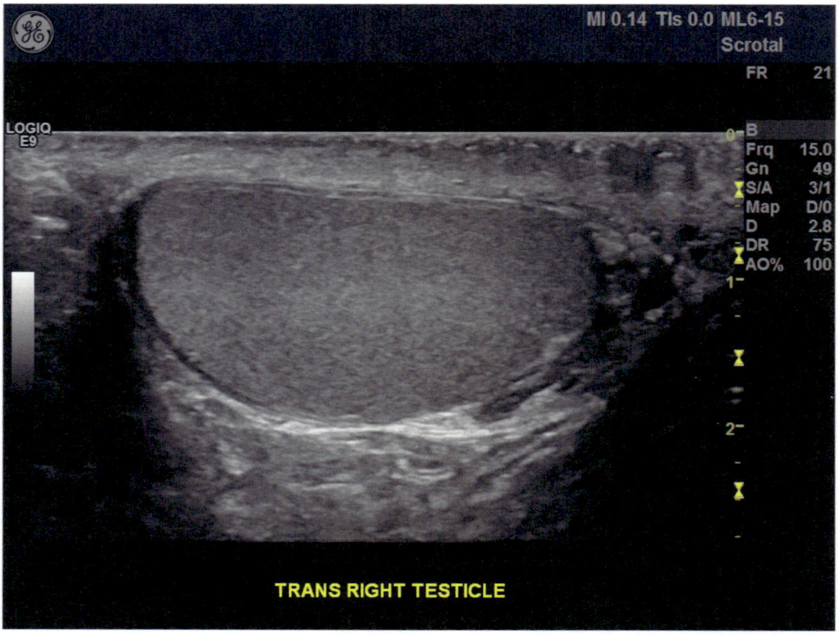

TRV right testicle

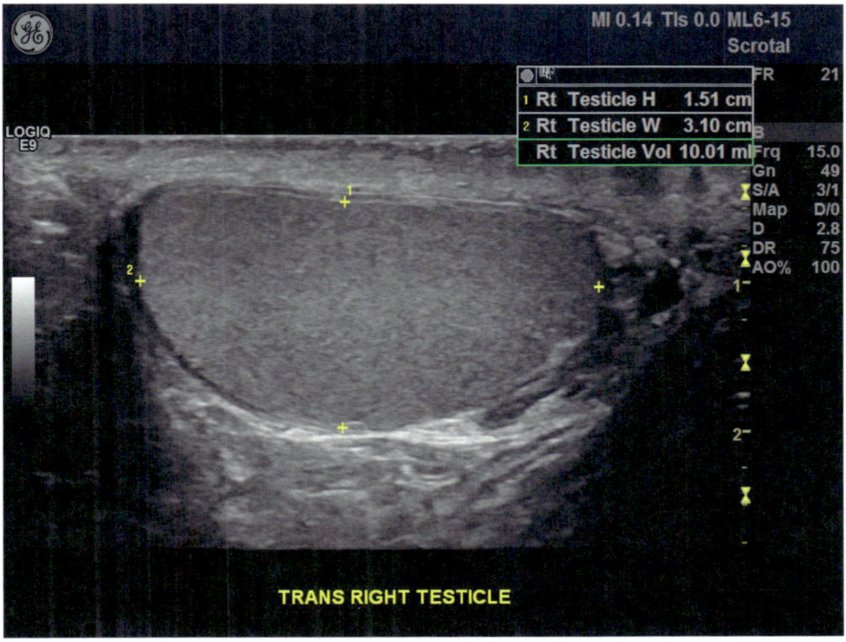

TRV right testicle with measurements

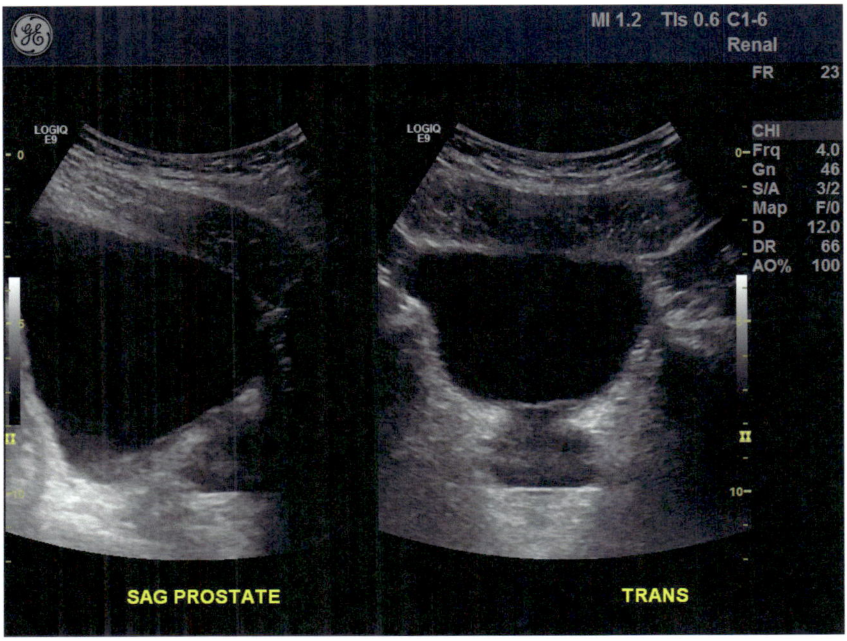

SAG + TRV prostate

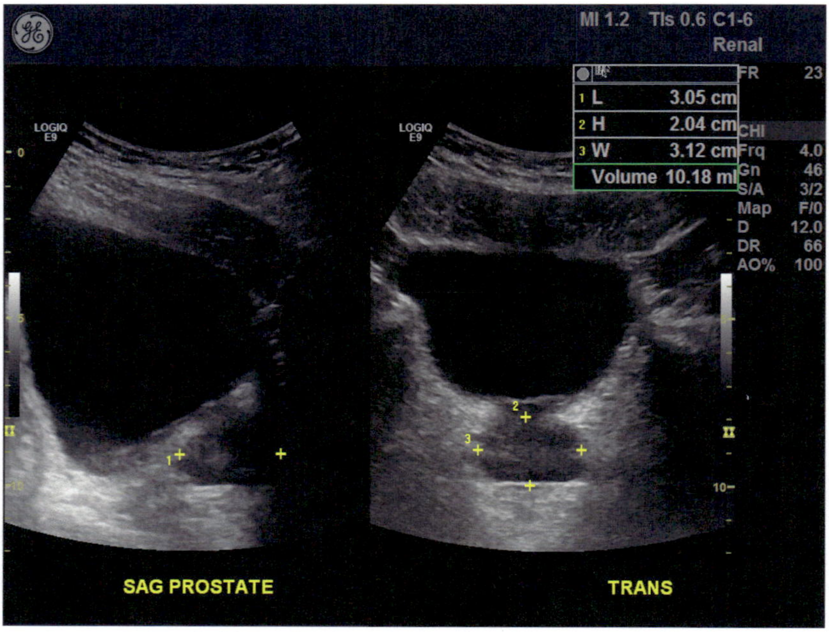

SAG + TRV prostate with measurements

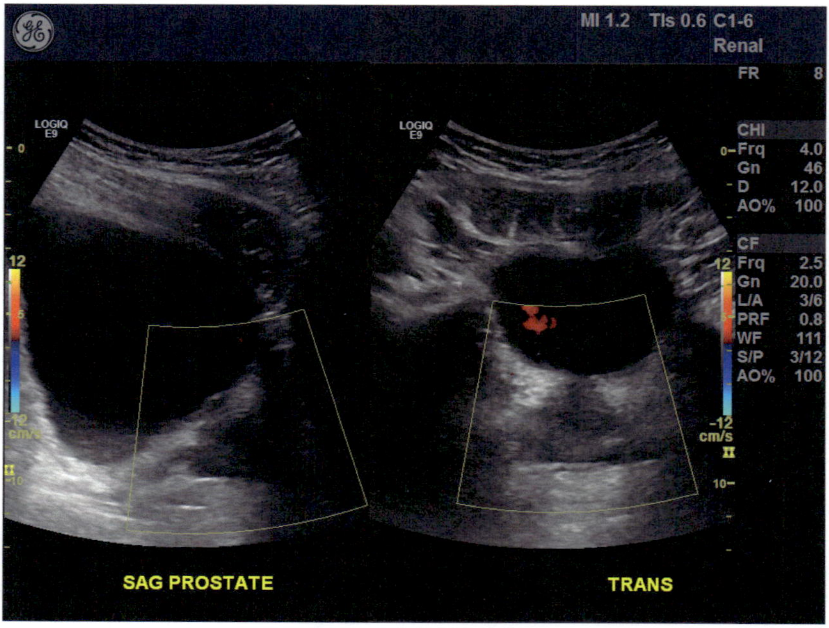

SAG + TRV prostate evaluated with color Doppler

Protocols

Scrotum:

1. TRV Buddy image
   a. 2D
   b. Color Doppler
   c. Measure the scrotal wall if it is edematous: AP
2. SAG RT EPI Head
   a. 2D
   b. Measurements: L + AP
   c. Color Doppler
3. TRV RT EPI Head
   a. 2D
   b. Measurements: W
   c. Color Doppler
4. SAG RT EPI Body + Tail
   a. 2D
   b. Color Doppler
5. SAG RT Testicle
   a. 2D
   b. Measurements: L + AP
   c. 2D: Med
   d. 2D: Lat
   e. Color Doppler
   f. Spectral Doppler (at both med/lat locations)
6. TRV RT Testicle
   a. 2D: Sup
   b. Mid
      i. 2D
      ii. Measurements: W
   c. 2D: Inf
7. Eval the lat scrotum for varicoceles

Do the same protocol for the left side when done with the right

Thyroid

Patient Prep and Exam

No patient prep.

Transducers Used

- Linear ML6-15
- Linear 9L

Exam Indications

- Goiter
- Hyperthyroidism
- Hypothyroidism
- Follow-up nodules

Functions and Labs

Structure:	Function:	Labs:
Parathyroid	Secretes PTH Regulates calcium and phosphate levels	PTH
Thyroid	Secretes 3 hormones (T3, T4, and calcitonin) Controls metabolism	TSH T3 T4

Normal Measurements

Structure:	Abbreviation/Acronym:	Measurements:
Parathyroid Gland		<0.5 x 0.3 x 0.1cm (Not normally seen on US unless abnormal - which the measurements will be larger)
Isthmus	ISTH	<1cm
Thyroid	THY	L: 4-6cm H: 2-3cm W: 1.5-2cm

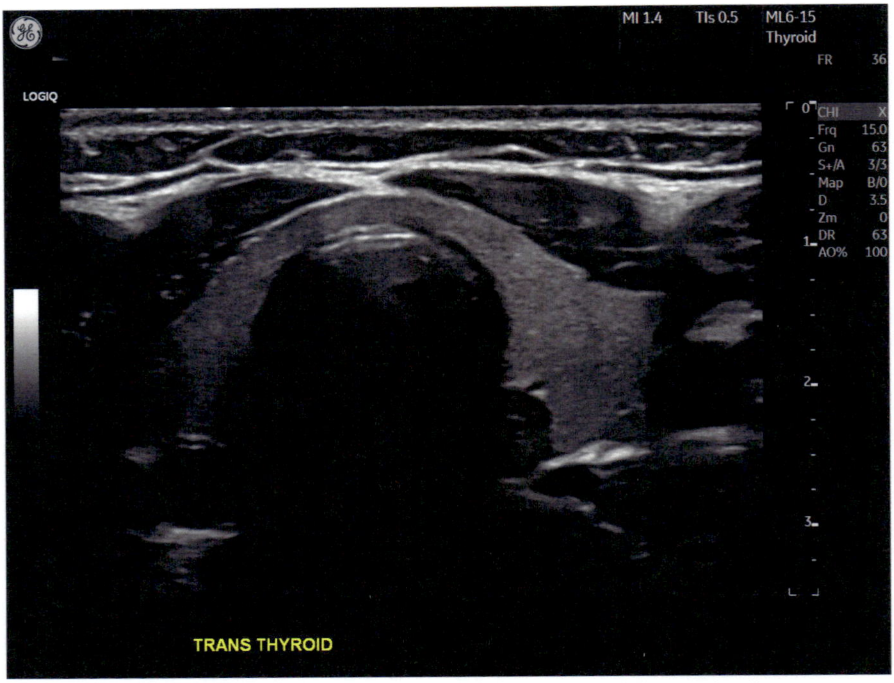

TRV thyroid midline showing the right and left lobes and isthmus

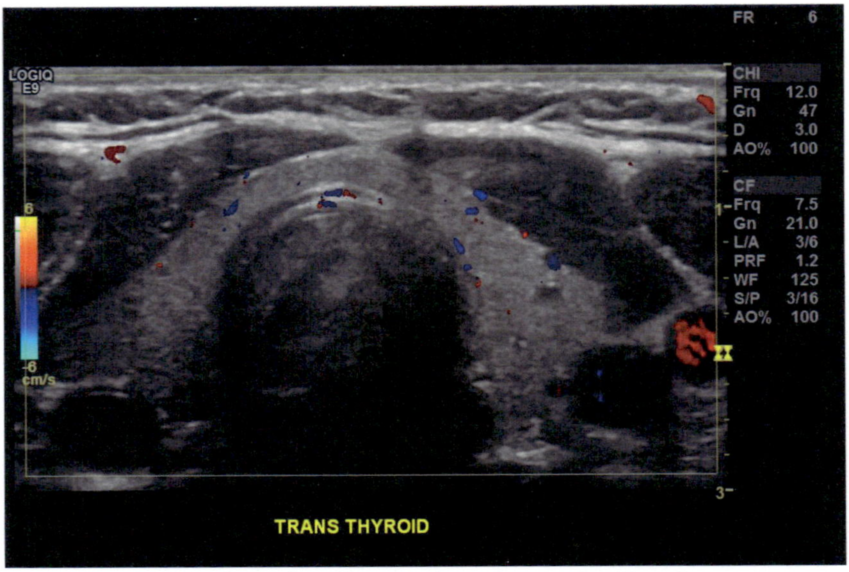

TRV thyroid midline evaluated with color Doppler

Helpful Tips

Don't be afraid to use the 9L transducer! The thyroid can sometimes live low in the neck where the clavicle gets in the way of the transducer, or the patient's neck can be a little larger. Use the 9L transducer for this! The 9L has deeper tissue penetration and can help you reach a deep thyroid.

Don't let the patient talk or chew gum during the exam. Talking and chewing gum causes vibrations, thus creating blurry images. It also causes flash artifact during color Doppler, making the thyroid or nodules look hyperemic. This results in a false diagnosis about blood flow.

If the patient is a fast or heavy breather, have them hold their breath or ask them to take shallow or slower breaths. Fast respirations also cause blurry images and flash artifact during color Doppler.

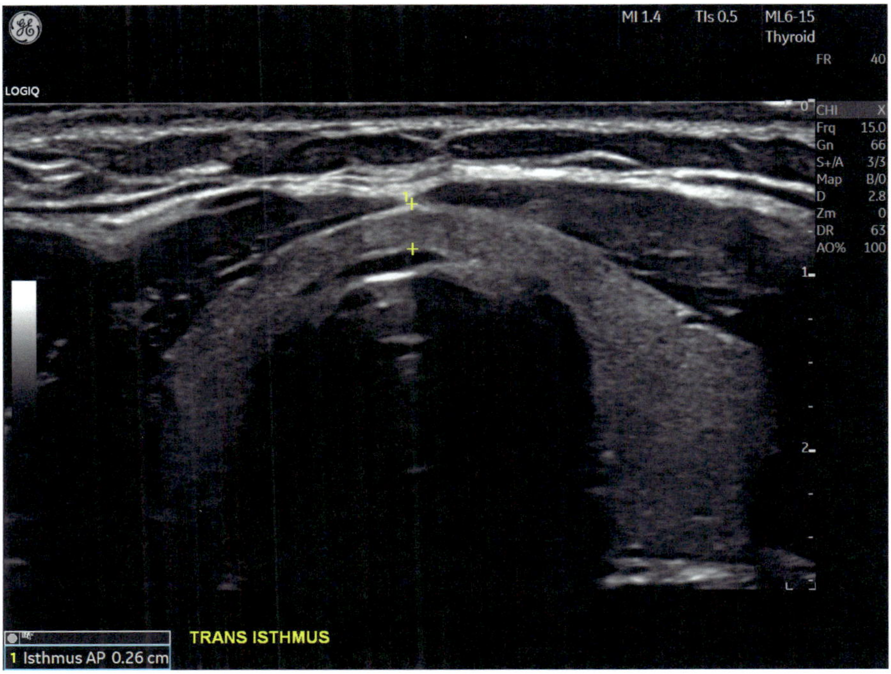

TRV isthmus with measurement

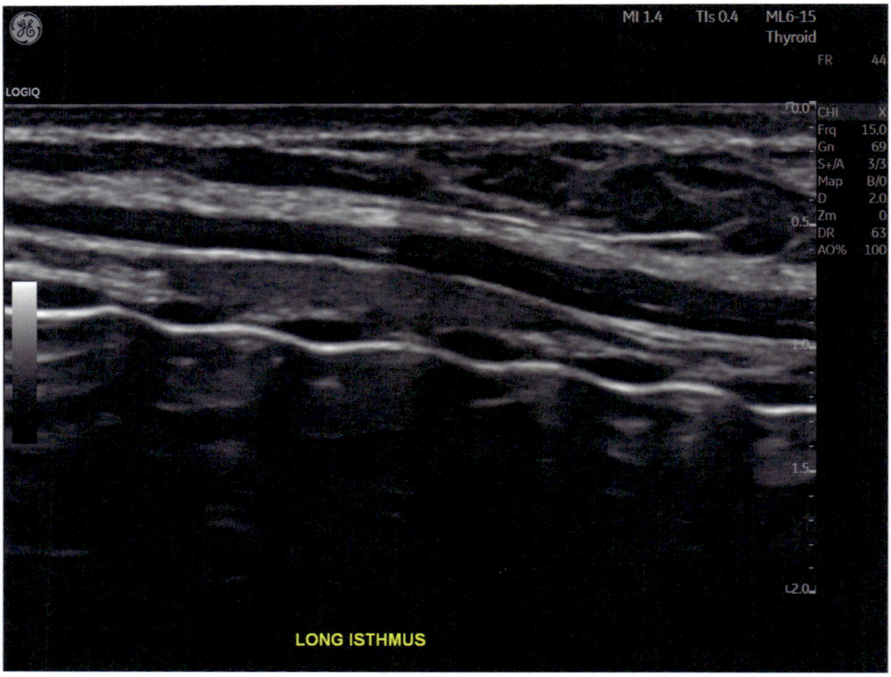
MI 1.4
TIs 0.4
ML6-15
Thyroid
FR 44
LOGIQ
CHI X
Frq 15.0
Gn 69
S+/A 3/3
Map B/0
D 2.0
Zm 0
DR 63
AO% 100
0.0
0.5
1.0
1.5
2.0
LONG ISTHMUS

SAG isthmus

TI-RADS:

Composition		Echogenicity		Shape		Margin		Echogenic Foci	
Cystic or almost completely cystic	**0 pts**	Anechoic	**0 pts**	Wider-than-tall	**0 pts**	Smooth	**0 pts**	None or large comet-tail artifacts	**0 pts**
Spongiform	**0 pts**	Hyperechoic or isoechoic	**1 pt**	Taller-than-wide	**3 pts**	Ill-defined	**0 pts**	Macro-calcifications	**1 pt**
Mixed cystic + solid	**1 pt**	Hypoechoic	**2 pts**			Lobulated or irregular	**2 pts**	Peripheral calcifications	**2 pts**
Solid or almost completely solid	**2 pts**	Very hypoechoic	**3 pts**			Extra thyroidal extension	**3 pts**	Punctate echogenic foci	**3 pts**

0 pts	**2 pts**	**3pts**	**4-6 pts**	**7+pts**
Benign	Not Suspicious	Mildly Suspicious	Moderately Suspicious	Highly Suspicious
No FNA	No FNA	Follow if ≥ 1.5cm FNA if ≥ 2.5cm	Follow if ≥ 1cm FNA if ≥ 1.5cm	Follow if ≥ 0.5cm FNA if ≥ 1cm

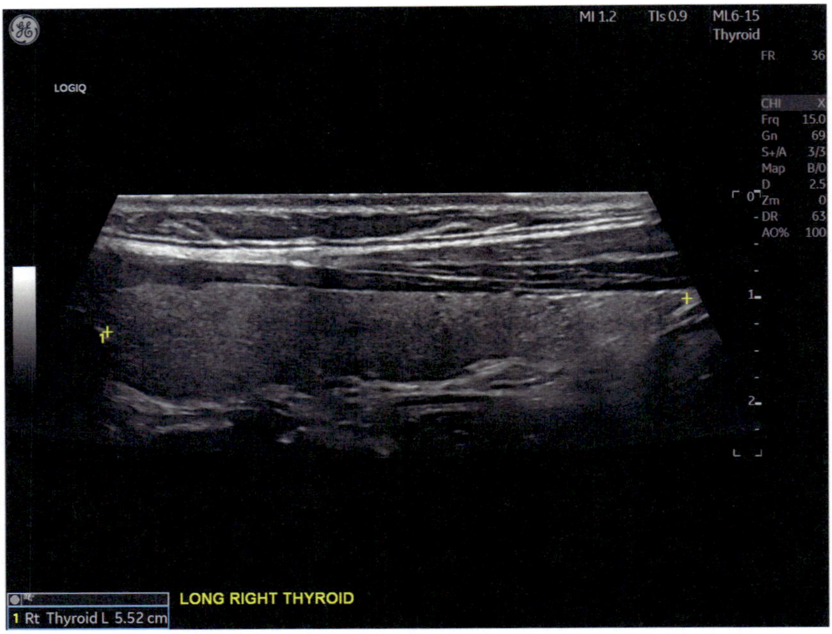

SAG right thyroid with measurement

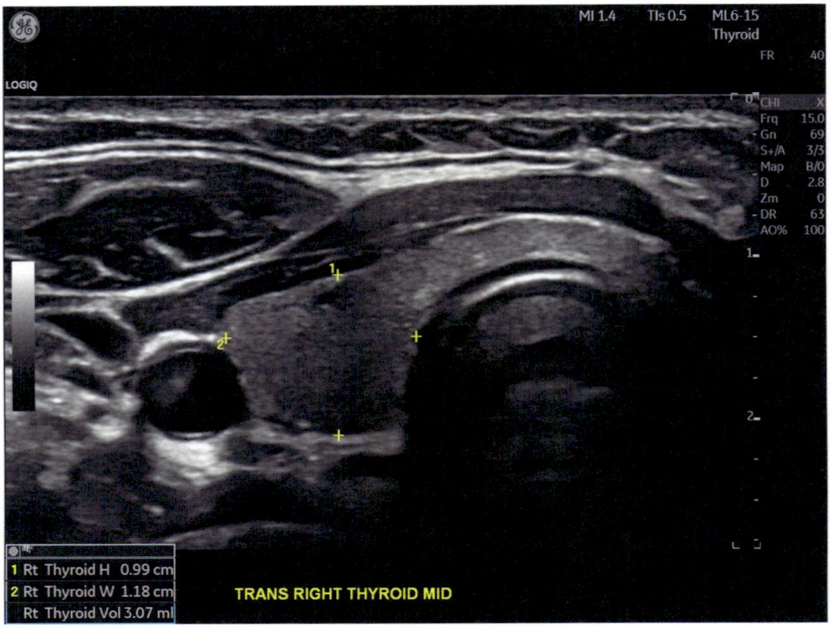

TRV right thyroid with measurements

Protocols

Thyroid:

1. TRV ML (show RT + LT lobes and isthmus)
2. TRV Isthmus
    a. 2D
    b. Measurements: AP
3. TRV RT Thyroid
    a. 2D: Sup
    b. Mid
        i. 2D
        ii. Measurements: AP + W
        iii. Color Doppler
    c. 2D: Inf
4. SAG RT Thyroid
    a. 2D
    b. Measurements: L
    c. Color Doppler
    d. 2D: Med
    e. 2D: Lat

Do the same protocol for the left side when done with the right

Notes

Notes

Notes

8

Vascular

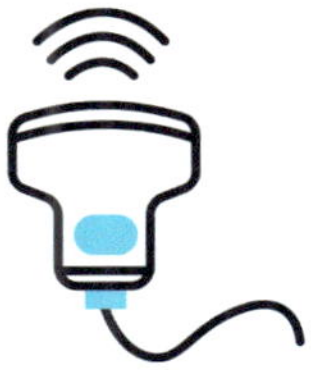

THIS CHAPTER INCLUDES VASCULAR exams that would be performed by an RVT in a general ultrasound department, NOT a vascular lab. Vascular labs have different protocols than we do in general labs. Our protocols and criteria may overlap; however, they are not uniform throughout all facilities. The following exams will be written out for a general department.

For information on the aorta, please see *Chapter 1: Abdomen* for information.

Carotid

Patient Prep and Exam

No patient prep.

Transducers Used

- Linear 9L

Exam Indications

- Vertigo / syncope
- Bruit
- CAD
- TIA / stroke
- Pulsatile neck mass

Normal Measurements

Structure:	Abbreviation /Acronym:	Measurement:	Velocity (cm/s):	Resistance:
Common Carotid Artery	CCA	-	Similar to ICA values	Low
External Carotid Artery	ECA	-	<115	High
Internal Carotid Artery	ICA	-	PS: <125 ED: <40	Low
Intima-Media Thickness	IMT	<0.8mm	-	-
Vertebral	VERT	-	20-60	Low

ICA Stenosis Grading

	PS (cm/s):	ED (cm/s):	ICA/CCA Ratio:
Normal	<125	<40	<2.0
<50% w/plaque	<125	<40	<2.0
50%-69%	125 - 230	40 - 100	2.0 - 4.0
>70%	>230	>100	>4.0
>80%	>230	>140	>4.0
Occluded (No Flow)	N/A	NA	N/A

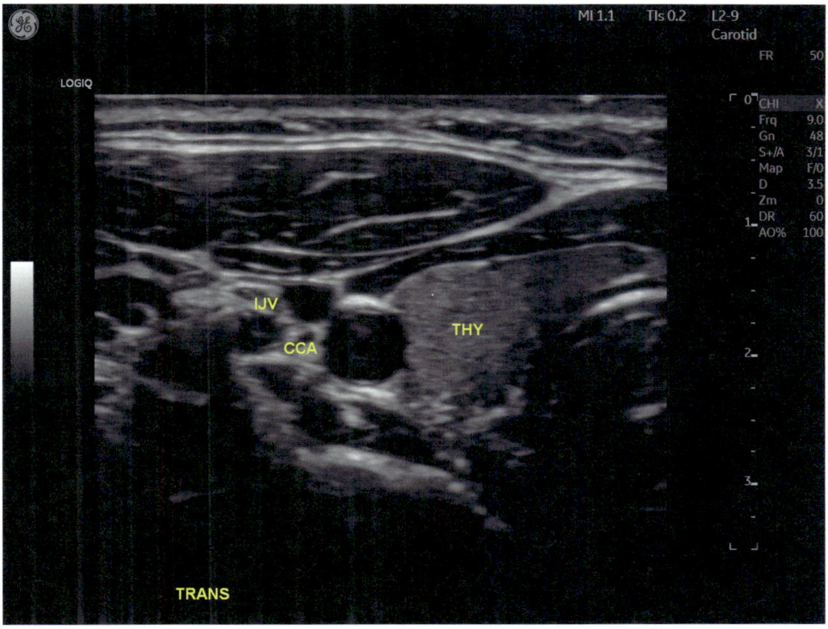

TRV right neck showing the location of the right CCA and IJV in comparison to the right thyroid lobe

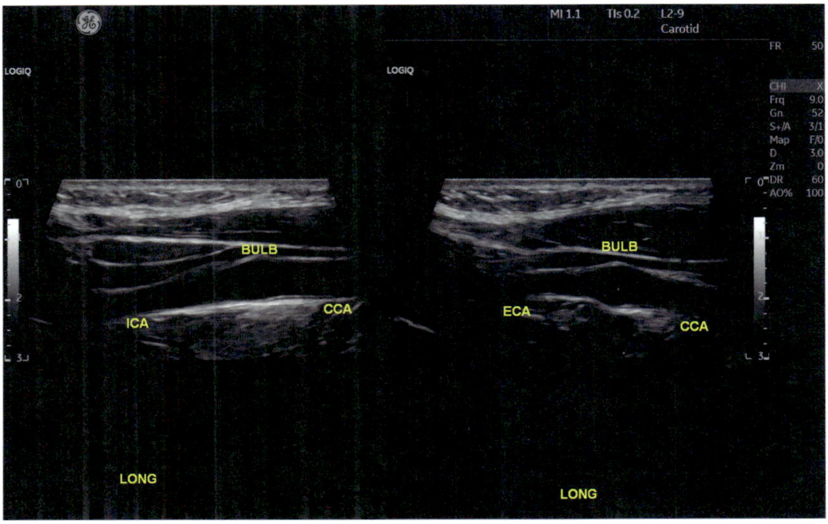

SAG bulb images with both the ICA and ECA

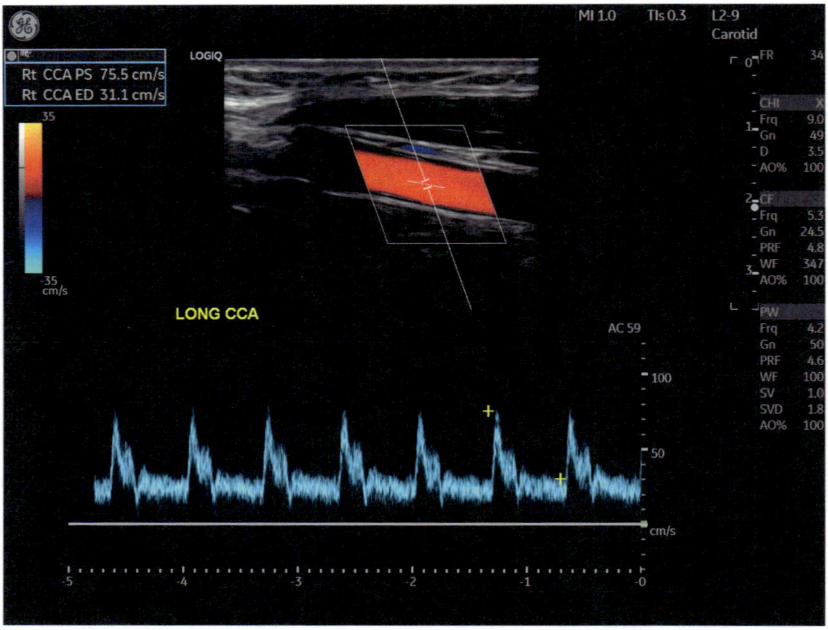

SAG CCA evaluated with color and spectral Doppler

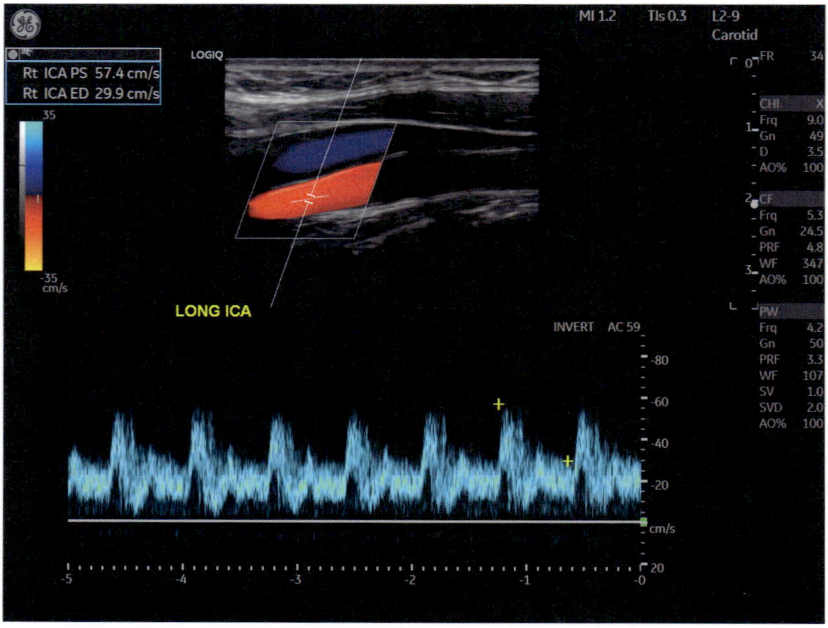

SAG ICA evaluated with color and spectral Doppler

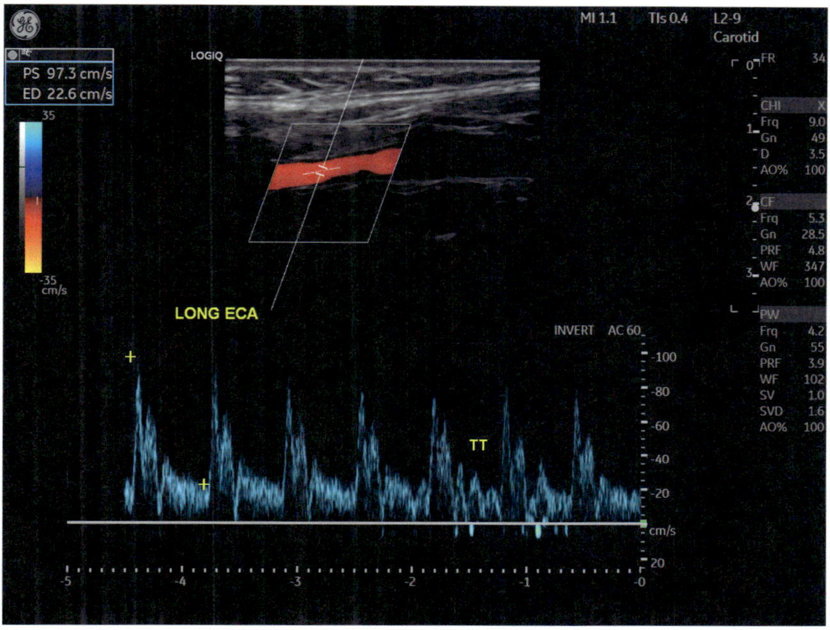

SAG ECA evaluated with color and spectral Doppler. The temporal tap was performed to signify that the ECA was evaluated and not the ICA

Something to keep in mind about the temporal tap is that it is considered a "soft" identifier. This is due to the oscillations that appear in the CCA and ICA. Also, the ECA and ICA can be in close proximity of one another, causing artifact and producing the temporal tap waveform on the ICA waveform. This can be confusing by making you think that you are in the ECA when you are really in the ICA.

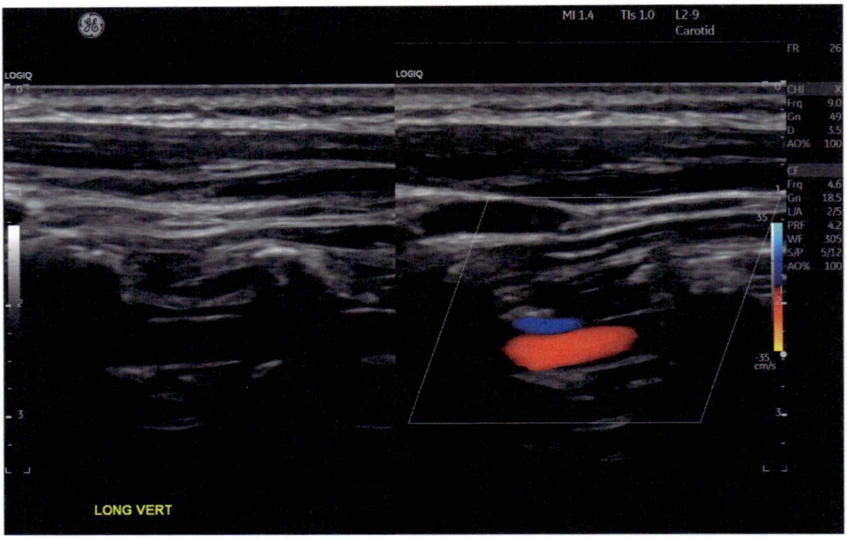

SAG vertebral artery evaluated with color Doppler

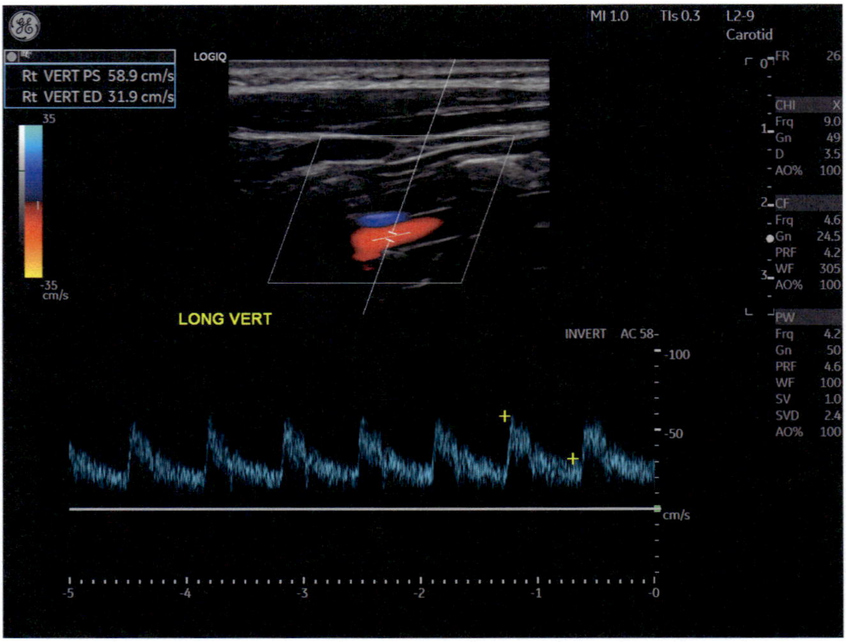

SAG vertebral artery evaluated with color and spectral Doppler

Protocols

Carotid:

1. TRV RT CCA
   a. 2D: P + M + D
2. TRV RT BIF
   a. Color Doppler
3. SAG RT CCA
   a. 2D: P + M + D
4. SAG RT BULB
5. SAG RT ICA
   a. 2D: P + M + D
6. SAG RT ECA
7. SAG RT CCA

Evaluate in 2D first. Pay attention to how much plaque and the kind of plaque that is in the arteries

Same protocol for the left side

8. SAG RT CCA
   a. P + M + D
      i. Color Doppler
      ii. Spectral Doppler
9. SAG RT BULB
   a. Color Doppler
10. SAG RT ICA
    a. P + M + D
       i. Color Doppler
       ii. Spectral Doppler
11. SAG RT ECA
    a. Color Doppler
    b. Spectral Doppler + TT
12. SAG RT VERT
    a. Color Doppler
    b. Spectral Doppler
13. SAG RT SBLCV P
    a. Color Doppler
    b. Spectral Doppler

Mesenteric / Splanchnic Doppler

Patient Prep and Exam

The patient needs to be NPO for 8 hours prior to the exam. The reason for this is because when the patient is NPO, the SMA waveform presents as high-resistance. If the patient eats, the the SMA waveform presents as low-resistance. This occurs because the intestines require more blood flow for digestion. If the SMA waveform remains high-resistance after the patient eats, then this could indicate mesenteric ischemia. If the patient eats or drinks prior to this exam, then they will need to be rescheduled.

Transducers Used

- Curvilinear C1-6

Exam Indications

- Post-prandial (post-po) pain
- Unexpected weight loss
- Post-surgical observation

Normal Measurements

Structure:	Abbreviation/ Acronym:	Velocities:	Resistance
Celiac Artery	CA	98 - 105cm/s	Low
Inferior Mesenteric Artery	IMA	74 - 200cm/s	**NPO:** High Resistance **PO:** Low Resistance
Superior Mesenteric Artery	SMA	PSV: 97 - 142cm/s EDV: <45cm/s	**NPO:** High Resistance **PO:** Low Resistance

Diagnostic Criteria

% Diameter Reduction	PSV (cm/s)
<70%	Celiac: <200 SMA: <275
71 - 99%	Celiac: >200 SMA: >200
Occluded	-

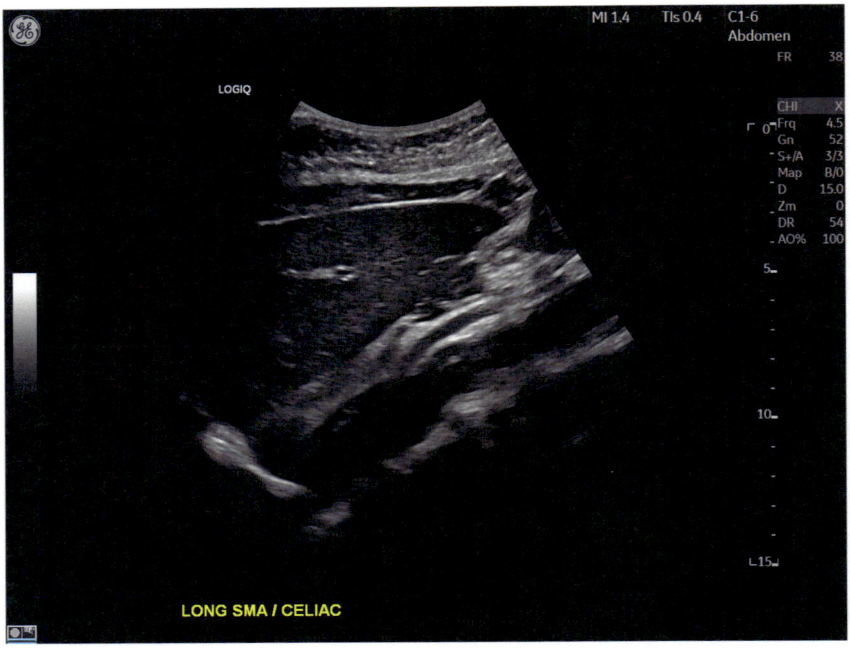

SAG SMA and celiac artery

Protocols

Celiac/SMA:

1. SAG AO
   a. P + M + D
      i. 2D
      ii. Color Doppler
      iii. Spectral Doppler
2. SAG AO (at the level of the celiac artery)
   a. Color Doppler
   b. Spectral Doppler
3. CHA
   a. Color Doppler
   b. Spectral Doppler
4. Splenic A
   a. Color Doppler
   b. Spectral Doppler
5. Celiac A
   a. P + D
      i. 2D
      ii. Color Doppler
      iii. Spectral Doppler
6. SMA
   a. Origin + P + M + D
      i. 2D
      ii. Color Doppler
      iii. Spectral Doppler
7. IMA P
   a. 2D
   b. Color Doppler
   c. Spectral Doppler

Don't forget to document any plaque in the aorta!

Liver Doppler

Patient Prep and Exam

The patient needs to be NPO for 8 hours prior to their exam.

Transducers Used

- Curvilinear C1-6

Exam Indications

- Cirrhosis
- Abnormal lab values (LFTs)
- TIPS (Transjugular Intrahepatic Portosystemic Shunt)
- PHTN (Portal Hypertension)

Notes!

What is a TIPS? A TIPS is a shunt that is connected from the portal vein to a hepatic vein. This shunt helps bypass blood that would otherwise flow through the liver. This helps patients that suffer from portal hypertension in cases of liver failure by reducing the pressure in the portal vein. This procedure does not cure liver failure, but it does help relieve some of the complications associated with it.

Normal Measurements

Structure:	Abbreviation /Acronym:	Measurements:	Velocities:	Notes:
Common Hepatic Artery	CHA		RI: 0.5 - 0.7	Hepatopetal (red color doppler) Low Resistance
Hepatic Veins	HVs			Hepatofugal (blue color doppler) Multiphasic
Liver	LIV	<18cm		
Main Portal Vein	MPV	AP: <13mm L: 8cm	15 - 39cm/s	Hepatopetal (red color doppler) Above baseline waveform on spectral Phasic with respirations

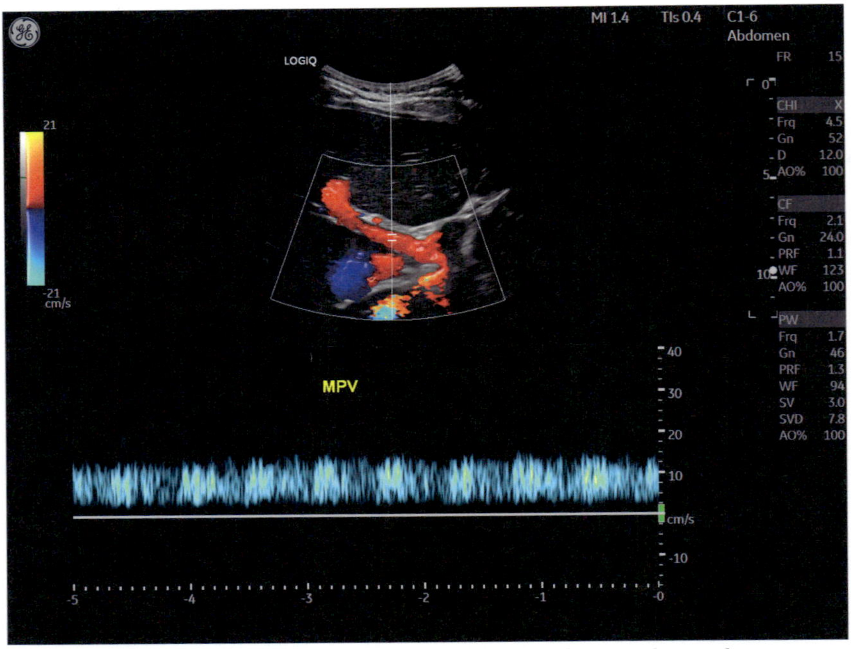

Main portal vein evaluated with color and spectral Doppler

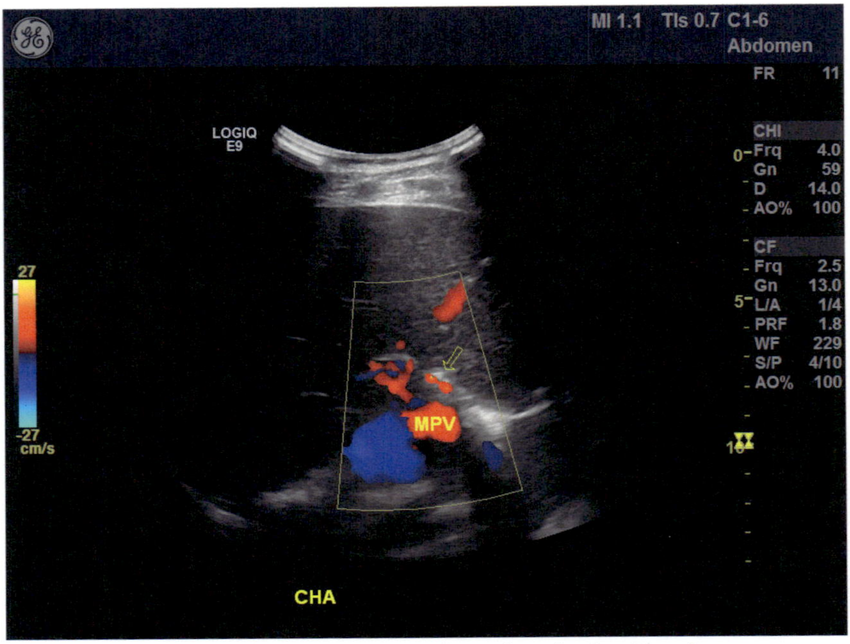

Common hepatic artery evaluated with color Doppler

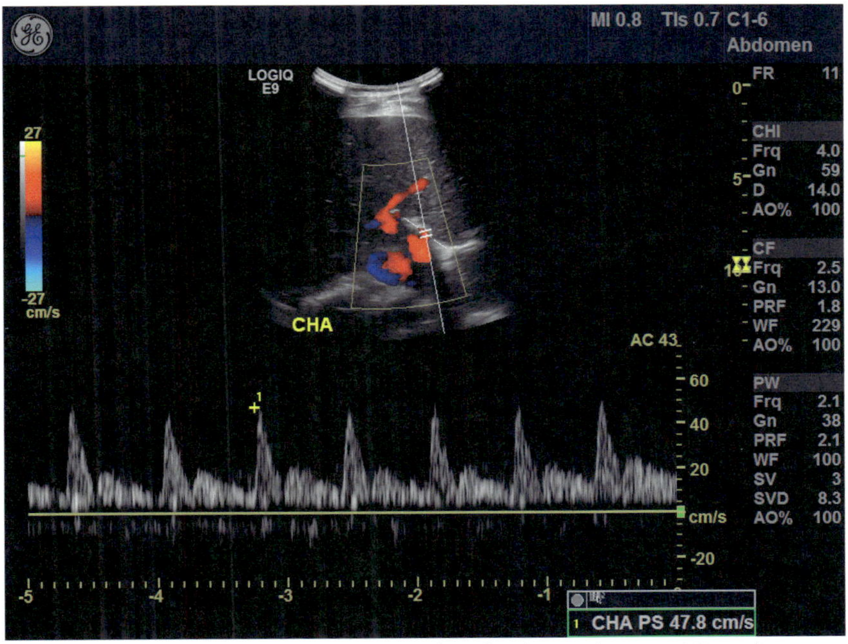

Common hepatic artery evaluated with color and spectral Doppler

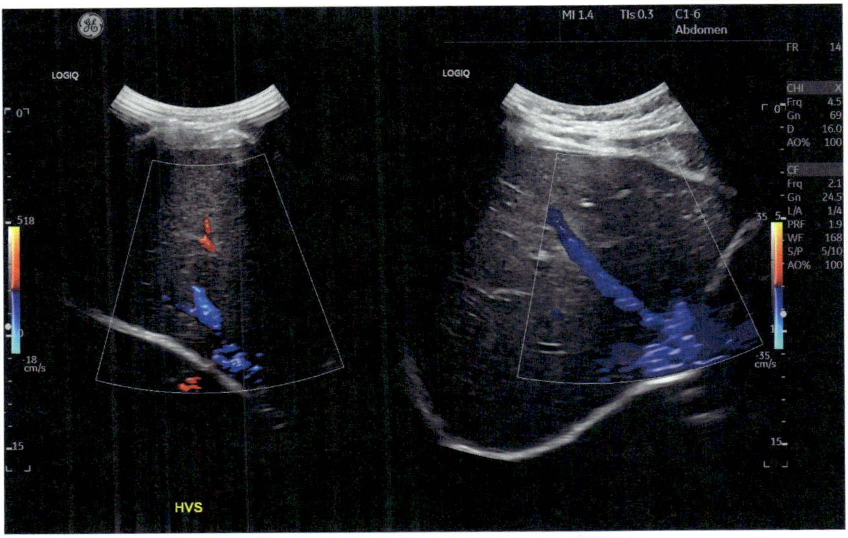

Hepatic veins evaluated with color Doppler

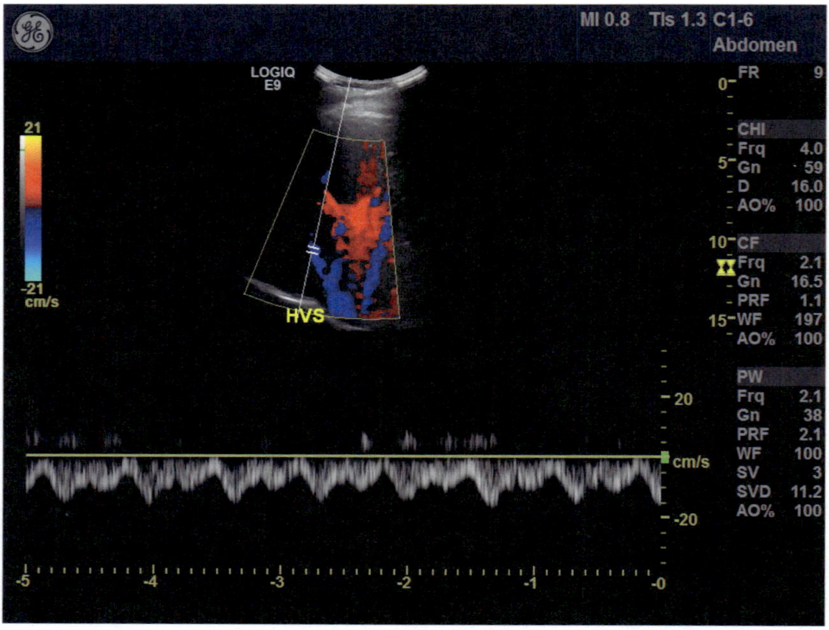

Hepatic vein evaluated with color and spectral Doppler

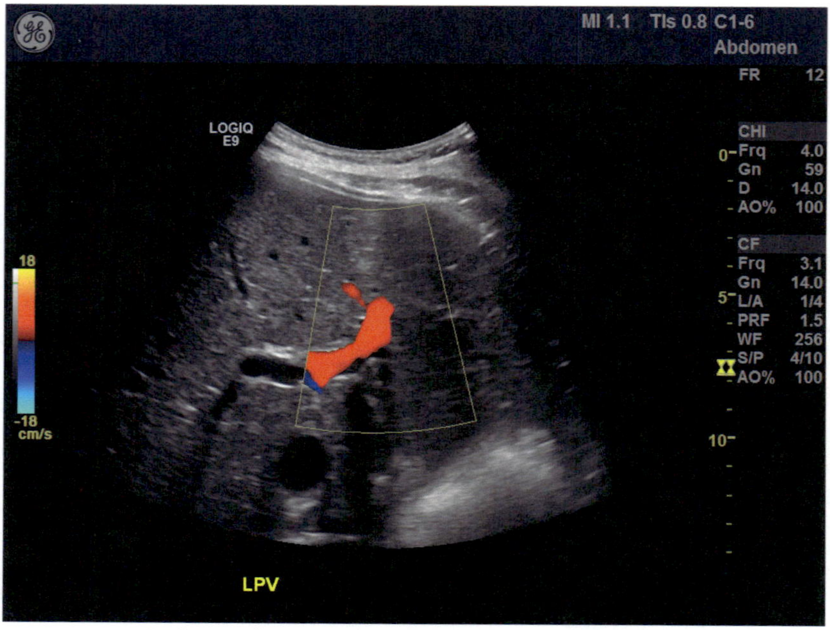

Left portal vein evaluated with color Doppler (red)

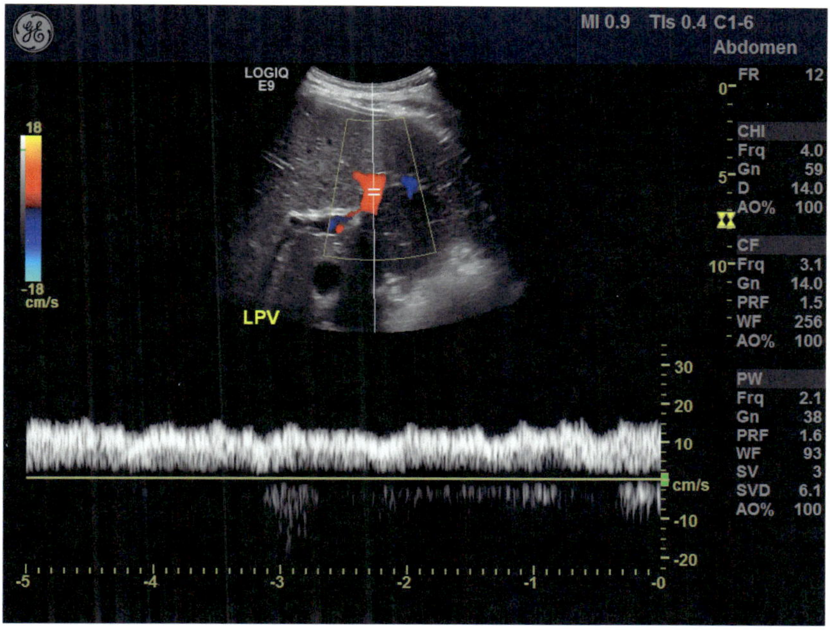

Left portal vein evaluated with color Doppler (red) and spectral Doppler

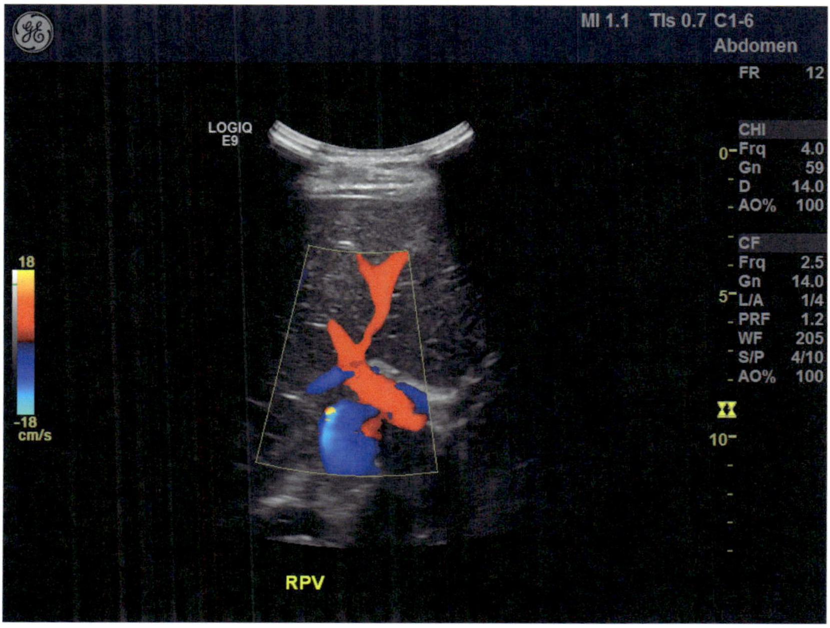

Right portal vein evaluated with color Doppler (blue)

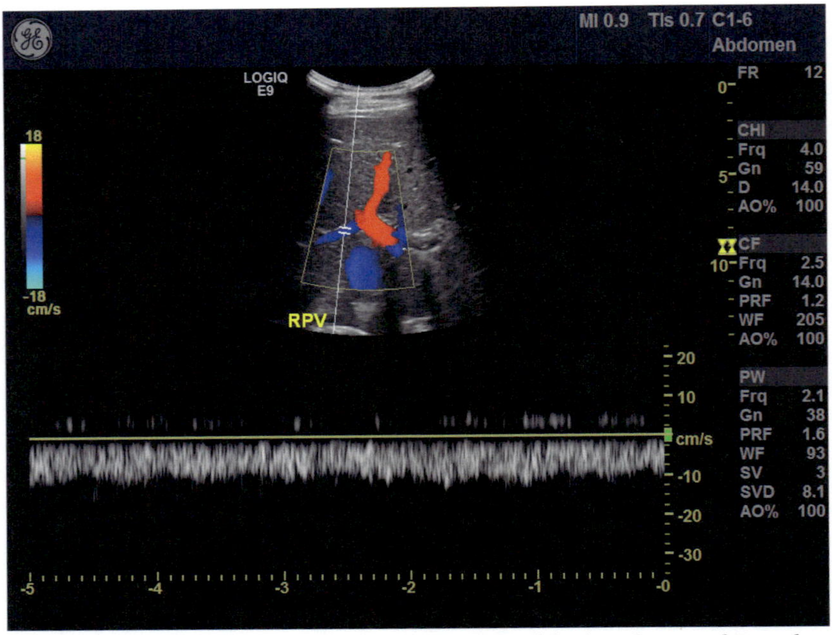

Right portal vein evaluated with color Doppler (blue) and spectral Doppler

Protocols

Liver Doppler:

1. SAG Liver
   a. 2D: Subcostal/Intercostal
   b. Measurements: L (with the RK in the image)
2. TRV Liver
   a. 2D: Subcostal/Intercostal
   b. Liver capsule (Linear ML6-15 transducer)
3. CHA
   a. Color Doppler
   b. Spectral Doppler
4. MPV
   a. Measurements: AP
   b. Color Doppler
   c. Spectral Doppler
5. RPV
   a. Color Doppler
   b. Spectral Doppler
6. LPV
   a. Color Doppler
   b. Spectral Doppler
7. HVs
   a. LHV + MHV + RHV
      i. Color Doppler
      ii. Spectral Doppler

Take a liver capsule image with the Linear ML6-15 to show if there is any nodularity

Renal Doppler

Patient Prep and Exam

The patient needs to be NPO for 8 hours prior to the exam. Not all imaging facilities will have patient's be NPO however, you will be dealing with bowel gas.

Transducers Used

- Curvilinear C1-6

Exam Indications

- Malignant / Resistant / Uncontrolled HTN
- Follow-up on known RAS
- Increased creatinine

Normal Measurements

Structure:	Abbreviation/ Acronym:	Velocities:	Resistance
Renal Artery	RA	**Adults:** 60 - 140cm/s or <180cm/s **Pediatrics:** 74 - 127cm/s	Low

Measurements:	RI:	RAR:	AT:	PI:	S/D:
0.5cm	0.5 - 0.7	<3.5	<0.07s	0.7 - 1.4	0.26 - 0.4

RI and RAR Equations

$$RI = \frac{\text{Peak Systolic Velocity - End Diastolic Velocity}}{\text{Peak Systolic Velocity}}$$

RI:	Resistance:
<0.5	Abnormally low
0.5 - 0.7	Normal Low
>0.7	Increased / high

$$RAR = \frac{\text{Renal Artery Peak Systolic Velocity}}{\text{Aortic Peak Systolic Velocity}}$$

Renal Artery Stenosis Classification

RA Diameter Reduction:	PSV (cm/s):	RAR:
Normal	<180	<3.5
<60%	>180	<3.5
>60%	>180	>3.5
Occluded	-	-

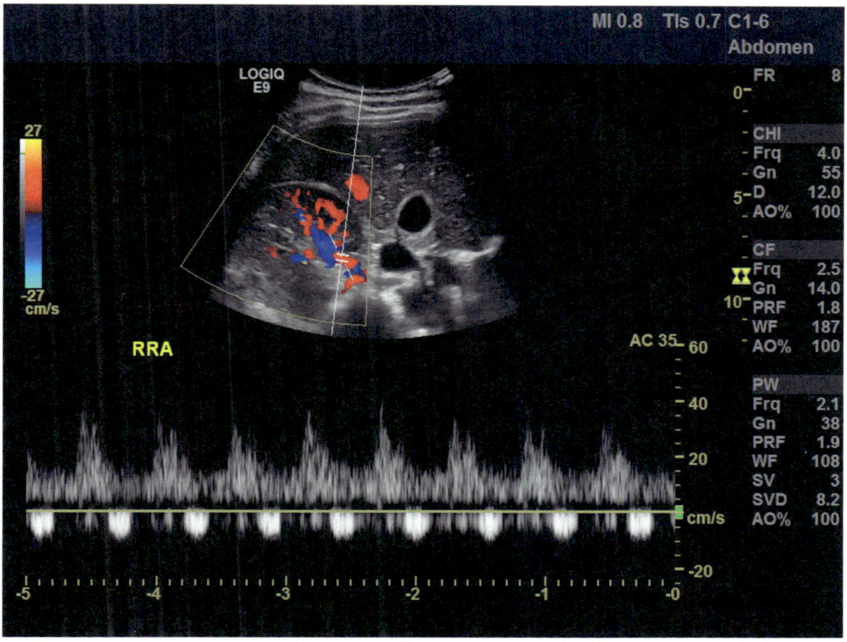

Right renal artery evaluated with color and spectral Doppler

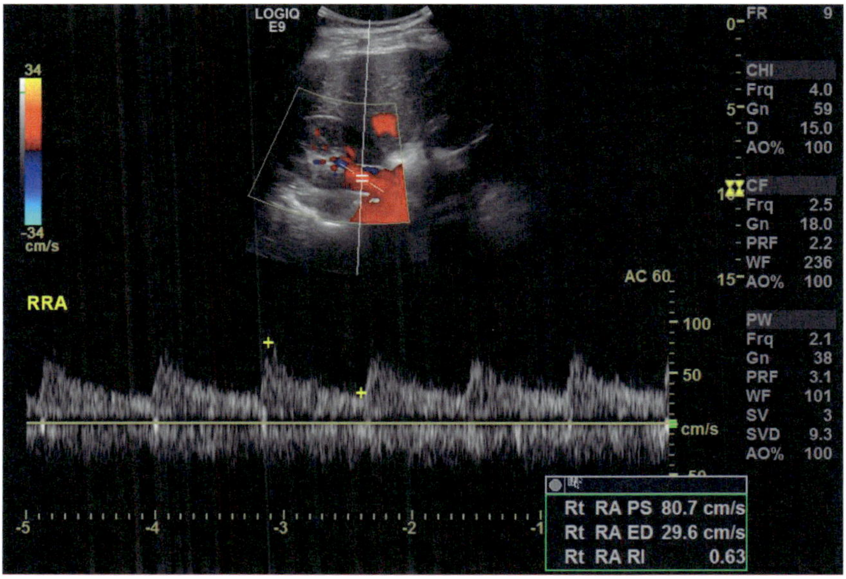

Right renal artery evaluated with color and spectral Doppler calculating an RI

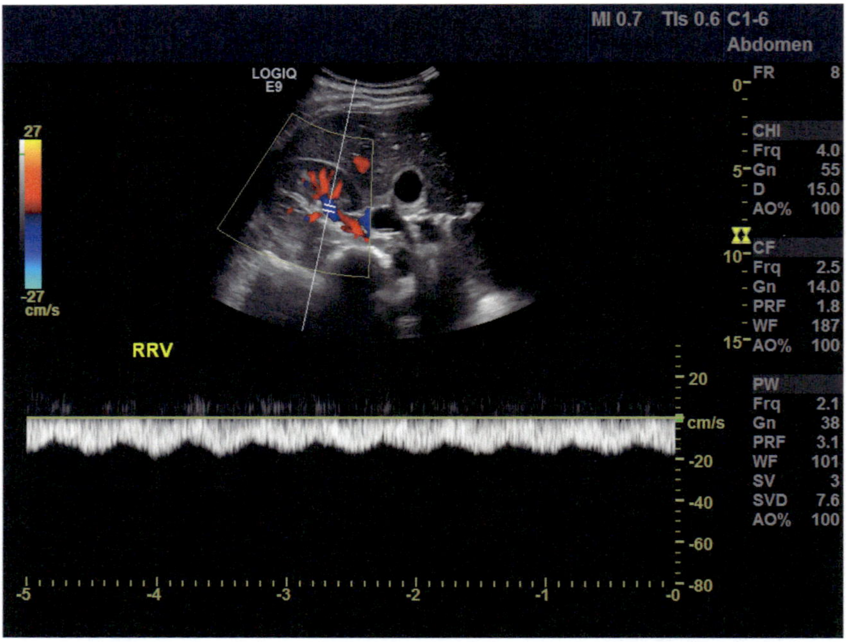

Right renal vein evaluated with color and spectral Doppler

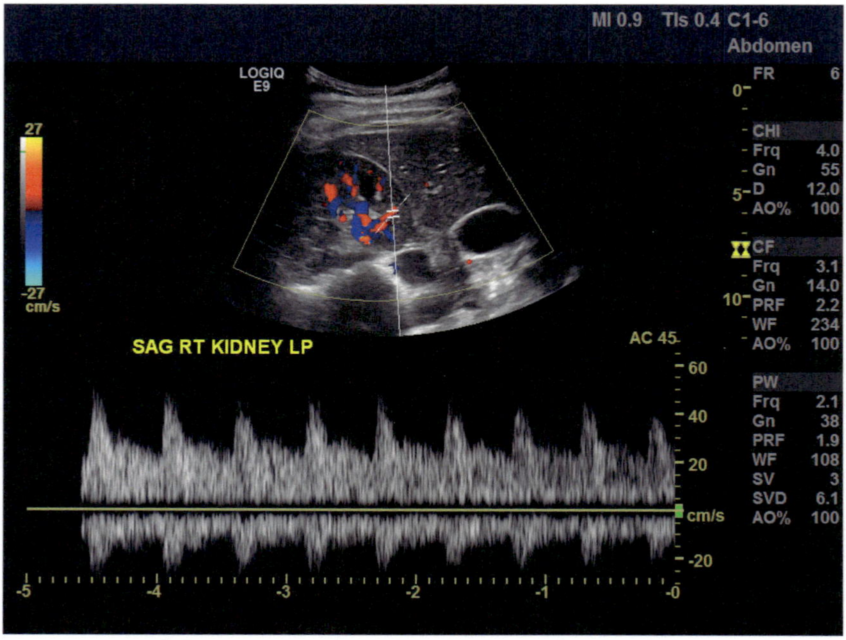

Interlobar artery evaluated with color and spectral Doppler

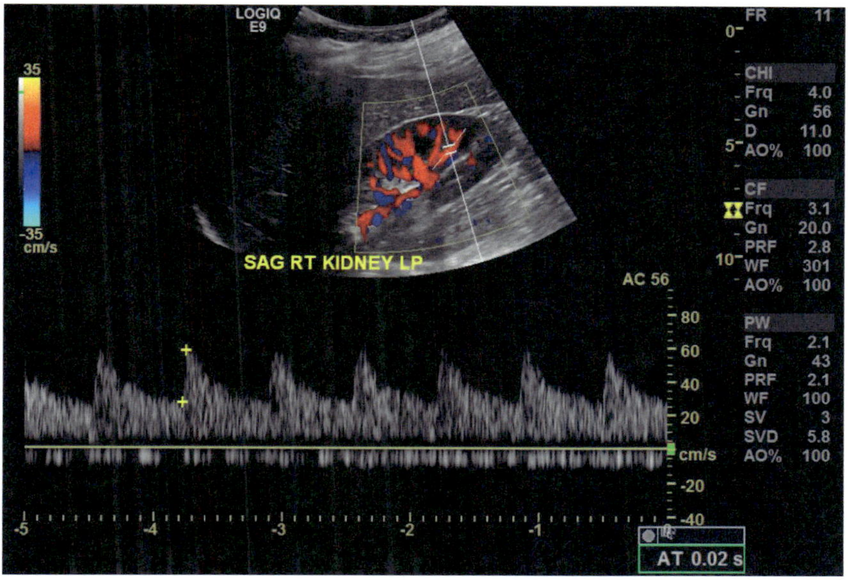

Interlobar artery evaluated with color and spectral Doppler calculating an AT

Protocols

Renal Doppler:

1. SAG AO
    a. P + M + D
        i. 2D
        ii. Measurements: AP
        iii. Color Doppler
2. SAG AO (level of the renal arteries)
    a. 2D
    b. Color Doppler
    c. Spectral Doppler
3. SAG RK
    a. 2D: ML
    b. Measurements: L
    c. Color Doppler
    d. 2D: M-L
4. TRV RK
    a. 2D: Sup
    b. Mid
        i. 2D
        ii. Measurements: AP + W
        iii. Color Doppler
    c. 2D: Inf
5. RRV
    a. Color Doppler
    b. Spectral Doppler
6. RRA
    a. Origin + P + M + D
        i. Color Doppler
        ii. Spectral Doppler
7. RT Interlobar Arteries
    a. Sup + Mid + Inf
        i. Color Doppler
        ii. Spectral Doppler

Do the same kidney protocol for the LK once done with the RK

Documentation will include PSV, EDV, RI, AT, and RAR

LEA + LEV

Patient Prep and Exam

No patient prep prior to the exam. When the patient arrives, they will need to remove their pants. If they wear long underwear, like boxers, those will need to be removed as well. A gown or blanket should be provided to keep the patient covered.

Transducers Used

- Linear 9L
- Curvilinear C1-6 (occasionally for larger legs or difficult calf veins)

ARTERIAL

Exam Indications

- Claudication
- Ischemic rest px
- PAD
- Arterial ulceration / Non-healing ulcer

Helpful Tips

Peripheral arteries are usually triphasic and high resistance, but not always. There have been many out there with biphasic waveforms that can be considered "normal". However, exercise causes vasodilation, producing hyperemic flow. Thus creating low resistance blood flow.

Normal Measurements

Structure:	Abbreviation/Acronym:	Velocity:
Anterior Tibial Artery	ATA	40-60cm/s
Common Femoral Artery	CFA	90 - 138cm/s
Dorsalis Pedis	DP	≈119cm/s
Deep Femoral Artery Profunda Femoris Artery Profunda	DFA PFA PROF	80-138cm/s
External Iliac Artery	EIA	100 - 140cm/s
Internal Iliac Artery	IIA	100-150cm/s
Peroneal	PERO	40-60cm/s
Popliteal	POP	50 - 80cm/s
Posterior Tibial Artery	PTA	40-60cm/s
Superficial Femoral Artery	SFA	Prox: 77 - 103 Dist: 79 - 107

Stenosis Grading

% Stensosis	Peak Velocity (cm/s)
Normal	<150
30-49%	150 - 200
50-75%	200 - 400
>75%	>400
Occluded	-

General labs don't typically take blood pressures and calculate ABIs (Ankle-Brachial Index). IAC accredited facilities should always be taking blood pressures and calculating ABIs. The equation and ABI criteria has been provided for reference.

A quick note about LEA exams and ABIs is that the arterial duplex exam only shows the presence of disease. It doesn't necessarily tell us how bad it really is. For example, there can be patients with femoral occlusions and only mild claudication.

ABIs on the other hand will give us information on the severity of disease. Therefore, vascular labs will perform ABIs and arterial duplex exams together. Some vascular labs will only do ABIs and will refrain from the arterial duplex if the results are normal. Some surgeons also prefer an angiogram over an arterial duplex, and therefore, it won't be done.

ABI:

$$\text{ABI} = \frac{\text{Ankle Systolic Pressure}}{\text{Brachial Systolic Pressure}}$$

Stage of Disease:	ABI:
Normal	1.0 - 1.3
Mild	0.9 - 1.0
Moderate	0.5 - 0.9
Mod-Severe	0.3 - 0.5
Severe	<0.3
Calcification/Vessel Hardening	>1.3

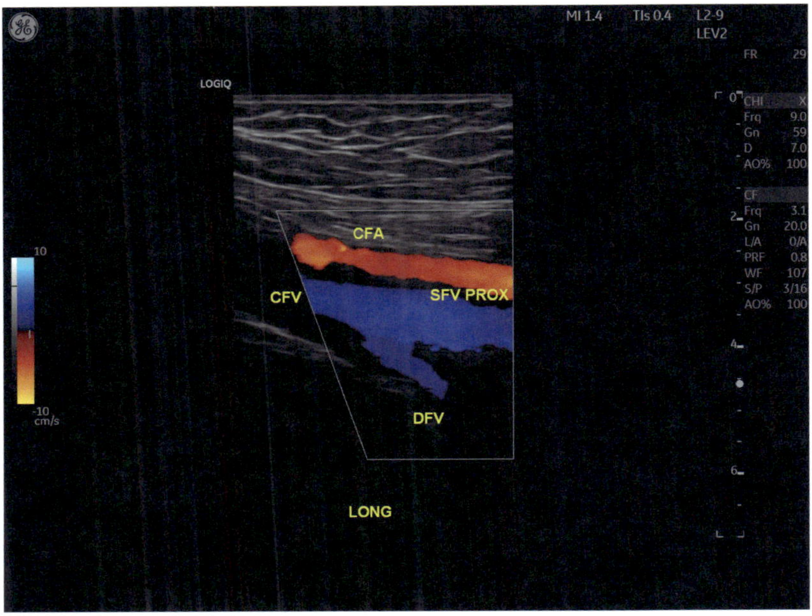

Showing the location of the CFA in comparison to it's vein counterpart

Protocols

Lower Extremity Arterial:

1. SAG CFA
2. SAG DFA

3. SAG SFA P
4. SAG SFA M
5. SAG SFA D

6. SAG POP P
7. SAG POP D

8. SAG ATA P
9. SAG ATA M
10. SAG ATA D

11. SAG PTA P
12. SAG PTA M
13. SAG PTA D

14. SAG PERO P
15. SAG PERO M
16. SAG PER D

17. SAG DPA

For every part of the protocol, you will take 3 images:

1. 2D
2. Color Doppler
3. Spectral Doppler

Don't forget to label what leg you are doing!

VENOUS:

Exam Indications

- Acute px
- Acute swelling
- SOB (Shortness of breath)

Helpful Tips

Things to keep in mind for a regular LE exam ruling out a DVT:

- We don't measure the vein AP diameters. We only measure the GSV during a vein mapping. See the Vein Mapping section at the end of the chapter
- We do use color and spectral Doppler to show the direction of blood flow. We don't necessarily care about the velocity of the venous flow. However, there are exceptions if there is a concern for venous stenosis caused by extrinsic compression or venous stent obstruction
- Make sure to compress all the veins every 2cm or so from the groin all the way down to the ankle

Depending on what facility you work for or intern at, they may not evaluate all these veins.

LEV

Structure:	Abbreviation/Acronym:	Image Locations:
Common Femoral Vein	CFV	Proximal to the GSV
Greater Saphenous Vein	GSV	Prox
Femoral Vein Superficial Femoral Vein	FV SFV	Prox + mid + dist
Deep Femoral Vein Profunda Femoris Vein Profunda	DFV PFV PROF	Prox
Popliteal	POP	Prox + dist
Gastrocnemius Veins	GASTROC V GASTROCS	There are 2 veins located in the pop fossa just adjacent to the pop v document both mid
Posterior Tibial Veins	PTV	There are 2 veins Prox + mid + dist
Peroneal Veins	PERO	There are 2 veins Prox + mid + dist
Popliteal Fossa	POP FOSSA	Eval this area for possible Baker's cysts

Notes!

SFV (superficial femoral vein) is becoming old terminology, due to the confusion on status of deep vs superficial vein. FV (femoral vein) is becoming the new standard.

Some departments may document the SV (soleal vein). However, it is not very common in general departments as it is in vascular labs.

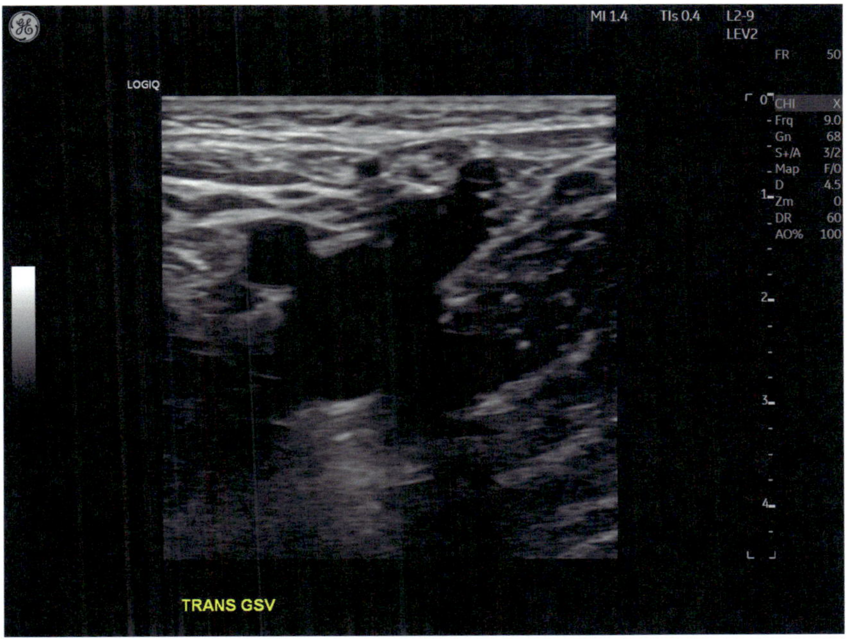

TRV GSV

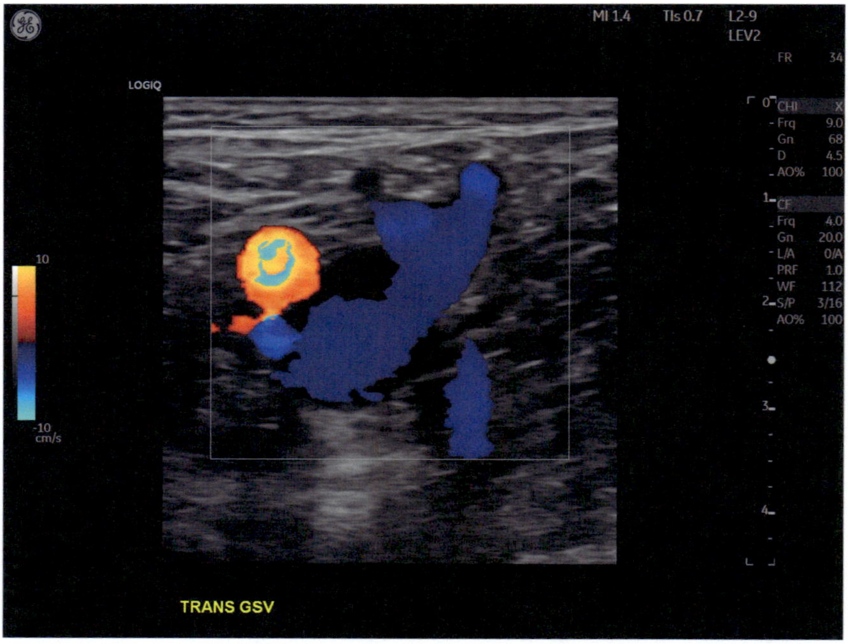

TRV GSV evaluated with color Doppler

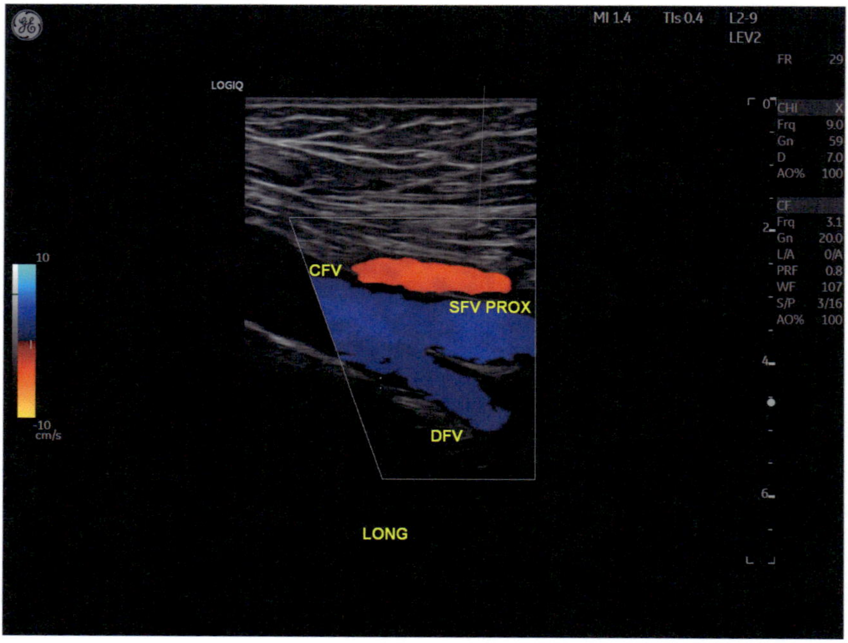

SAG CFV bifurcating into the SFV prox and DFV

Tips to get pesky calf veins!

Don't use all of these tricks at once. I typically will only change 2 things before I get adequate flow. Try them all out at some point in time and see what works for you and what you like best. I know a lot of people struggle with this, so here are some tips.

- Use the curvilinear transducer. This helps with penetration through larger calves and edema and is more sensitive to venous flow

- Position the patient into a steeper reverse Trendelenburg. This helps pool blood at the feet

- Hold the transducer at an angle on the patient's leg

- Use a warm blanket to wrap the calves before scanning them. This helps increase blood flow circulation

- Turn on "slow flow" or drop the color Doppler scale down to 5

- Set accumulation to 0.35. If you set it to less than that, the vessel may not fill nicely, and if you set accumulation above that, you are going to witness a lot of artifact and color bleed

- Set the threshold to 100%

- Use power Doppler

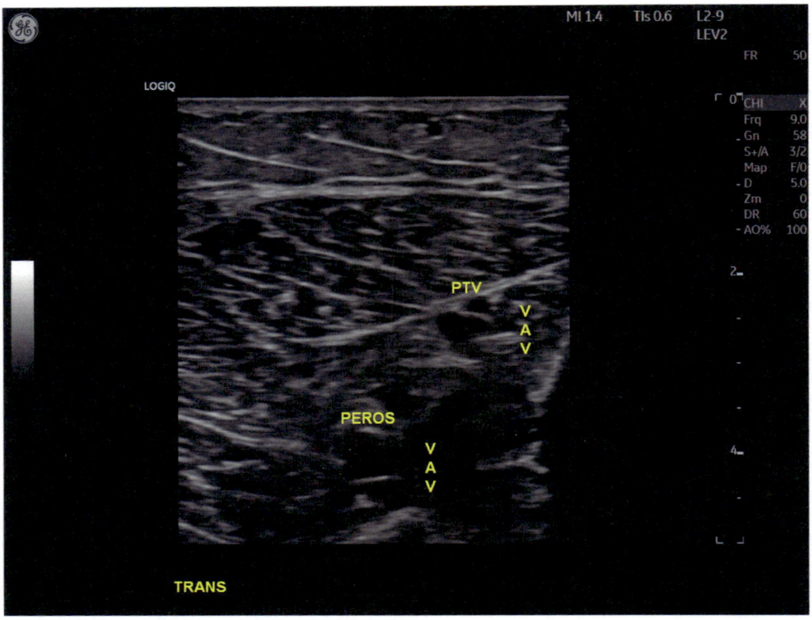

TRV PTVs and Peroneal veins. Annotated on right, veins and arteries on left. V: Vein A: Artery

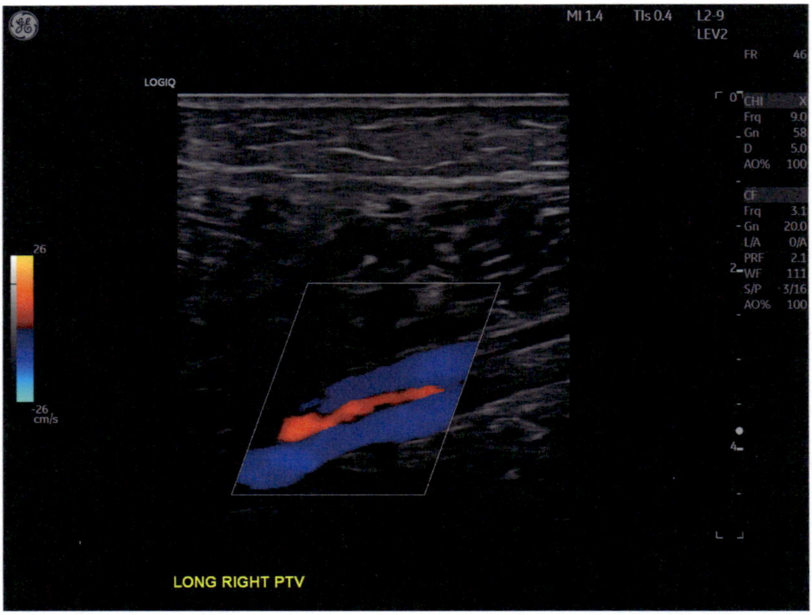

SAG right PTVs evaluated with color Doppler (blue). The PTA is red

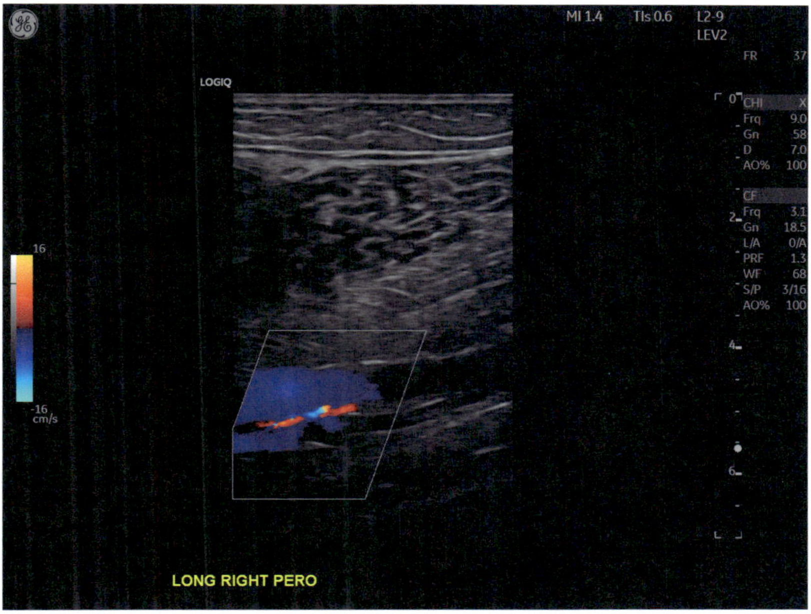

SAG right peroneal veins evaluated with color Doppler (blue). The Peroneal artery is red

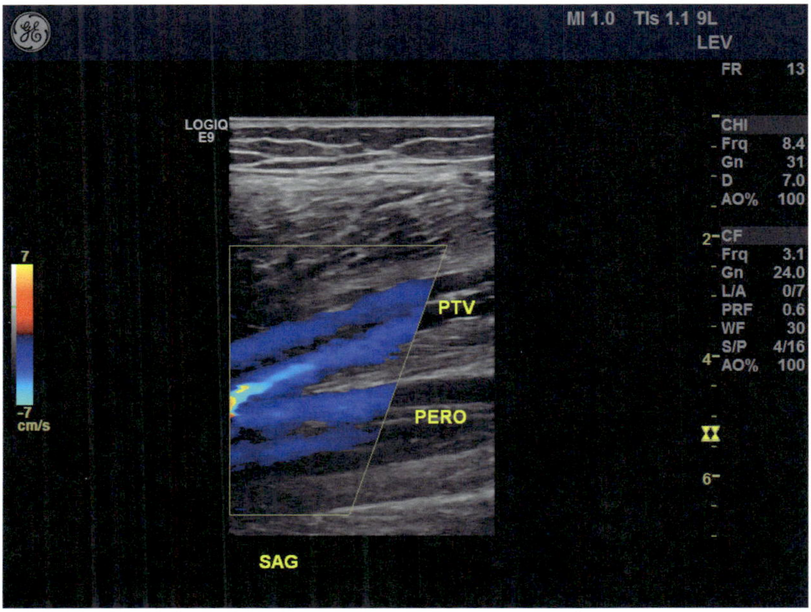

Both PTVs and peroneal veins are evaluated with color Doppler in the same image

Notes!

Steps 1-9 (the first half of this protocol) will be taken as 2D dual-screen images. The left side of the screen will be the TRV 2D non-compressed vein, and the right side of the screen will be the TRV compression image of that same vein. This is what rules out a DVT.

For the second half of this protocol, steps 10-14, take single-screen images. These images will be done in SAG and not TRV! Each step will have a color Doppler and spectral Doppler with augment image. Only augment if the patient is negative for DVT! If you augment on a patient that is positive for DVT, you could potentially dislodge the clot and send it to the lungs, giving the patient a PE (pulmonary embolism).

Steps 15-16 will also be done in single-screen, and will be done in SAG and not TRV! For these images, evaluate with color Doppler only and not spectral. Keep in mind that some departments will want spectral Doppler as well.

Protocols

Lower Extremity Venous:

1. TRV CFV
2. TRV GSV
3. TRV DFV
4. TRV SFV P
    a. P + M + D
5. TRV POP
    a. P + D
6. SAG POP Fossa (evaluate for a Baker's cyst)
7. TRV GASTROCS
8. TRV PTVs
    a. P + M + D
9. TRV PEROs
    a. P + M + D
10. SAG CFV
    a. Color Doppler
    b. Spectral Doppler w/augment
11. SAG GSV
    a. Color Doppler
    b. Spectral Doppler w/augment
12. SAG DFV
    a. Color Doppler
    b. Spectral Doppler w/augment
13. SAG SFV
    a. P + M + D
        i. Color Doppler
        ii. Spectral Doppler w/augment
14. SAG POP
    a. P + D
    b. Color Doppler
    c. Spectral Doppler w/augment
15. SAG PTVs
    a. P + M + D
        i. Color Doppler
16. SAG PEROs
    a. P + M + D
    b. Color Doppler

Compress the veins every 2cm, evaluating for clot

Only augment if the patient is negative for DVT!

UEA + UEV

Patient Prep and Exam

No patient prep prior to the exam. When the patient arrives, they will need to remove their shirt, and if they are wearing a bra, the strap will need to be off the shoulder and under the axilla. You may then give them a gown to keep them covered.

Transducers Used

- Linear 9L

ARTERIAL

Exam Indications

- Trauma
- Claudication
- Absent pulse
- Ulcer
- Pulsatile mass

Normal Measurements

Structure:	Abbreviation/ Acronym:	Measurements:	Velocities:
Axillary	AX	-	70 - 120cm/s
Brachial	BRACH	>2mm	50 - 100cm/s
Radial	RAD	-	40 - 90cm/s
Subclavian	SBCLV	-	70 - 120cm/s
Ulnar	ULN	-	40 - 90cm/s

Protocols

Upper Extremity Arterial:

1. SAG SBCLV P
2. SAG SBCLV D
3. SAG AX
4. SAG BRACH P
5. SAG BRACH M
6. SAG BRACH D
7. SAG RAD P
8. SAG RAD M
9. SAG RAD D
10. SAG ULN P
11. SAG ULN M
12. SAG ULN D

For every part of the protocol, you will take 3 images:

1. 2D
2. Color Doppler
3. Spectral Doppler

Don't forget to label what arm you are doing!

VENOUS

Exam Indications

- Acute px
- Acute swelling
- SOB

Helpful Tips

Things to keep in mind for a regular UE exam ruing out a DVT:

UEV studies have a lot of variability in protocol depending on where you work. For example some places will document the cephalic and basilic veins all the way from the proximal upper arm, down to the wrist. While others won't document those veins in the forearm at all. Another difference is that some places will document the radial and ulnar veins from the proximal to distal forearm, with compressions, color and spectral Doppler. While others only do compressions and one color picture. The reason for the variability is because these veins can become quite small and possibly not even visible with ultrasound.

When performing this study, just like the lower extremity venous study, we do evaluate with color and spectral Doppler. However, we don't necessarily care about the velocity of flow. We care more about the direction of flow and if there is clot that impedes it. The blood flow should be blue on color Doppler and be represented below the baseline on spectral Doppler.

Another thing to remember is that we do not measure the veins for this exam. If you are measuring veins, it would be for a vein mapping study. See the *Vein Mapping* section at the end of this chapter for more information.

UEV

Structure:	Abbreviation/Acronym:	Image Locations:
Internal Jugular Vein	IJV	Prox + mid + dist
Subclavian	SBCLV	Prox + dist
Axillary	AX	Mid
Cephalic	CEPH	Prox + mid + dist
Basilic	BAS	Prox + mid + dist
Brachial	BRACH	There are 2 veins Prox + mid + dist
Antecubital Fossa	AC FOSSA	This is a common site for clot due to being a highly used location for IV lines during hospital stays
Radial	RAD	There are 2 veins Prox + mid + dist
Ulnar	ULN	There are 2 veins Prox + mid + dist

Notes!

Some people augment for this exam and some don't. If you do augment, make sure to do the whole protocol in 2D with and without compression images first to rule out DVT. I will say this again; if you augment on a patient that is positive for DVT, you could potentially dislodge the clot and send it to the lungs, giving the patient a PE (pulmonary embolism). Once you are done with compression images, then you can go back and do color and spectral Doppler with augmentation only if the patient is negative for blood clot.

The 2D with and without compression images will be taken in dual screen. The left side of the screen will be an image of the open, non-compressed vein. The right side of the screen will be an image of the compressed vein.

Remember! There are two brachial, radial, and ulnar veins. In some patients, they will actually have three. You need to document all of them.

As I stated above, some departments will document the cephalic and basilic veins in the forearm. However, for simplicity, I am not going to include that in this protocol.

Protocols

Upper Extremity Venous:

1. TRV IJV
    a. P + M + D
        i. 2D with and w/o compression
2. SAG IJV
    a. P + M + D
        i. Color Doppler
        ii. Spectral Doppler
3. SAG SBCLV
    a. P + D
        i. Color Doppler
        ii. Spectral Doppler
4. TRV CEPH
    a. P + M + D
        i. 2D with and w/o compression
5. SAG CEPH
    a. P + M + D
        i. Color Doppler
        ii. Spectral Doppler
6. TRV AX
    a. 2D with and w/o compression
7. SAG AX
    a. Color Doppler
    b. Spectral Doppler

Compress the veins every 2cm, evaluating for clot

8. TRV BASIL
    a. P + M + D
        i. 2D with and w/o compression
9. SAG BASIL
    a. P + M + D
        i. Color Doppler
        ii. Spectral Doppler
10. TRV BRACH
    a. P + M + D
        i. 2D with and w/o compression
11. SAG BRACH
    a. P + M + D
        i. Color Doppler
        ii. Spectral Doppler
12. TRV AC Fossa
13. TRV RAD
    a. P + M + D
        i. 2D with and w/o compression
14. SAG RAD
    a. P + M + D
        i. Color Doppler
15. TRV ULN
    a. P + M + D
    b. 2D with and w/o compression
16. SAG ULN
    a. P + M + D
    b. Color Doppler

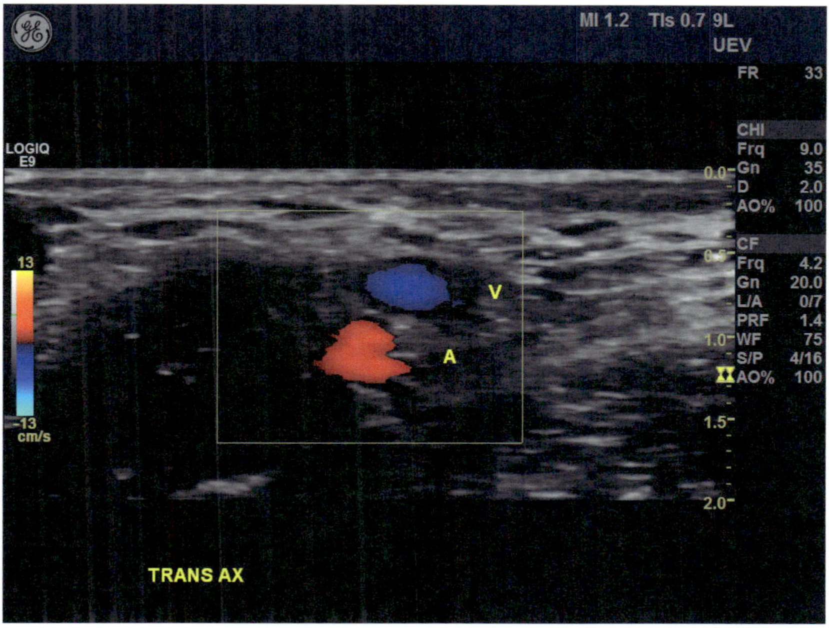

TRV axillary artery (red) and vein (blue)

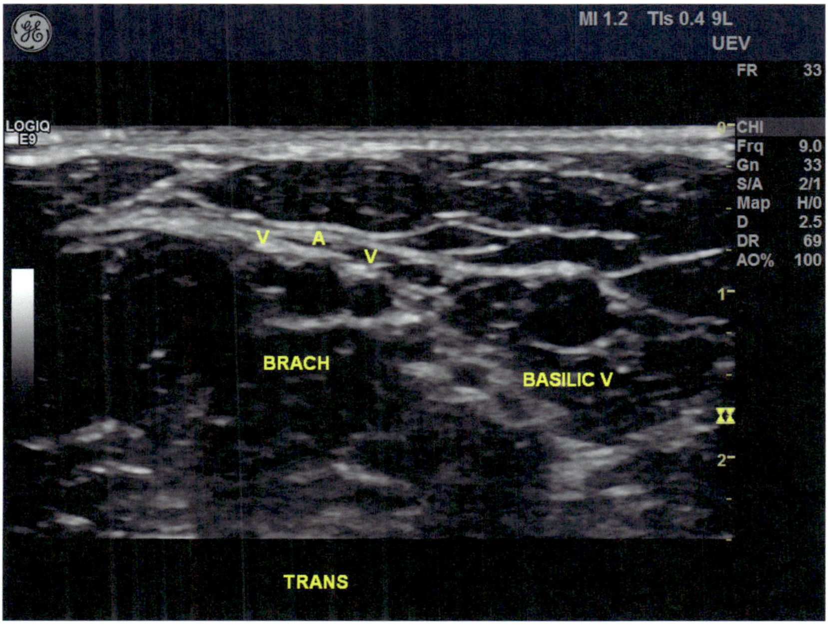

TRV brachial artery (A) and veins (V) lateral to the basilic vein

Notes!

Be careful to not mistaken the median nerve for an adjacent brachial vein, as it runs parallel to the brachial artery. Unfortunately this is a common mistake because the median nerve can emulate or bear resemblance to a brachial vein with clot due to it's heterogenous appearance and close proximity to the brachial artery.

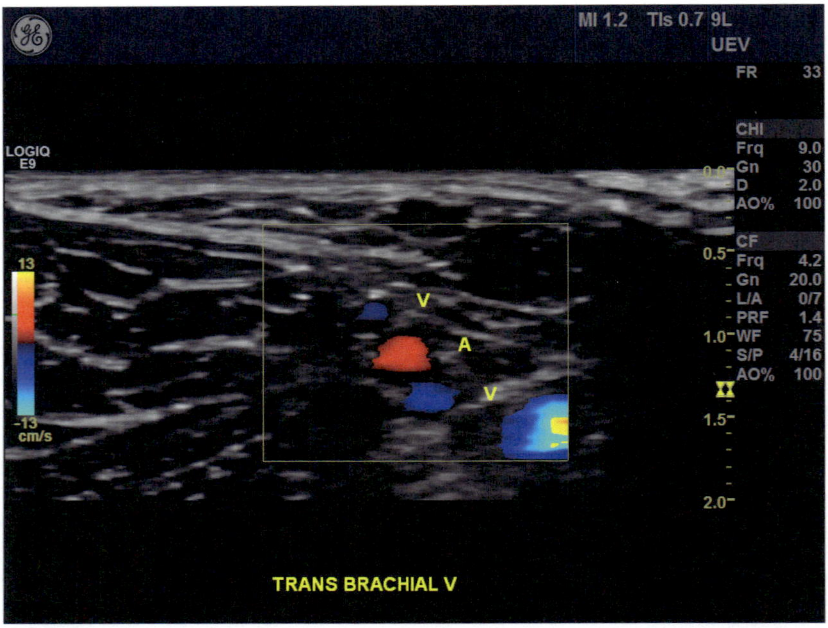

TRV brachial artery (red) and veins (blue) evaluated with color Doppler

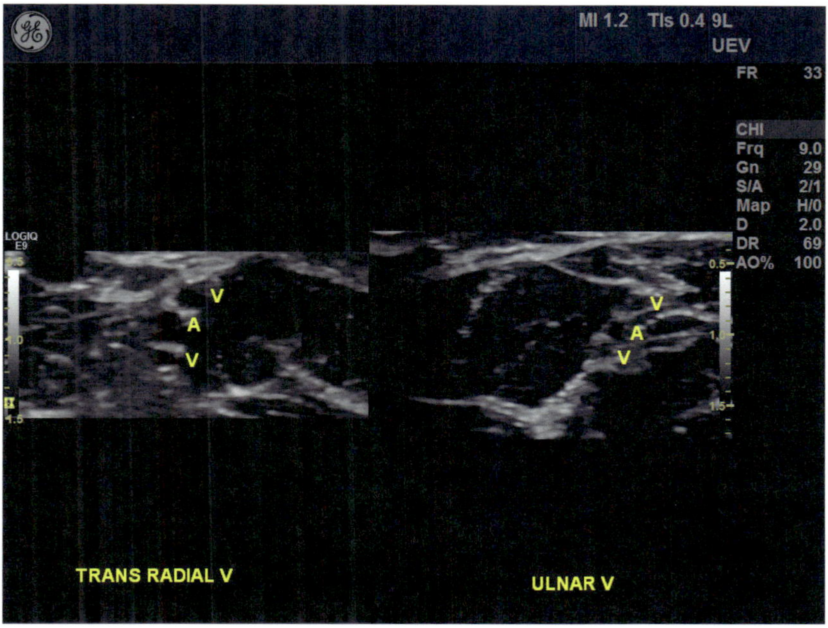

TRV radial artery (A) and veins (V) on the left. TRV ulnar artery (A) and veins (V) on the right

Vein Mapping

Patient Prep and Exam

Patient prep is different depending on the type of vein mapping exam being performed. Please refer below for the patient prep needed.

Transducers Used

- Linear 9L

Lower Extremity

Patient Prep and Exam

For this exam, the patient will need to remove their pants. If they wear long underwear, those will need to be removed as well. We need to have access to the whole leg from the groin down to the ankle.

Exam Indications

- Bypass graft
- Coronary artery bypass graft

Helpful Tips

For this exam, we only evaluate the GSV. The GSV must be a minimum of 2mm in AP diameter to be usable for revascularization. 2.5mm however, is more ideal.

Normal Measurements

Structure:	Abbreviation/Acronym:	Measurements:
Greater Saphenous Vein	GSV	Thigh: 4 - 6mm Calf: 2 - 3mm

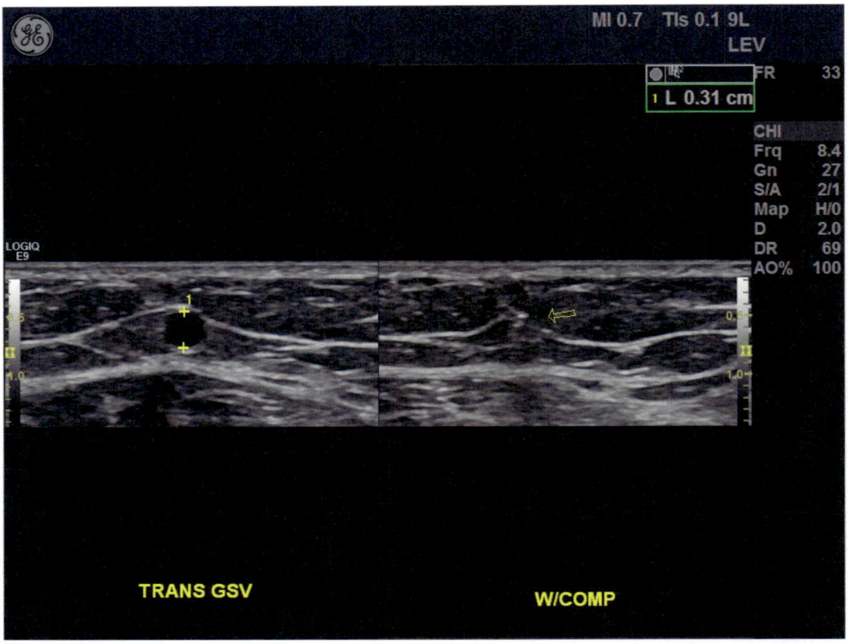

TRV GSV with measurement on left and compressed / fully collapsed GSV on right

Notes!

The first half of this protocol will be done in dual screen. The left side of the screen will be in TRV without compression, and the right side of the screen will be in TRV with compression. Take an AP measurement of the non-compressed vein on the left side of the screen. Document any and all evidence of obstruction. This refers to clot and intraluminal scarring.

Compress each vein every 2cm, evaluating for obstruction.

The second half of this protocol will be done in single-screen. We will evaluate the veins with both color and spectral Doppler.

Protocols

LE Vein Mapping

1. TRV GSV: Thigh
    a. P + M + D
        i. Take images with and without compression + AP measurement on the non-compressed vein
2. TRV GSV: Pop Fossa
    a. P + M + D
        i. Take images with and without compression + AP measurement on the non-compressed vein
3. TRV GSV: Calf
    a. P + M + D
        i. Take images with and without compression + AP measurement on the non-compressed vein
4. SAG GSV: Thigh
    a. P + M + D
        i. Color Doppler
        ii. Spectral Doppler w/ augment
5. SAG GSV: Pop Fossa
    a. P + M + D
        i. Color Doppler
        ii. Spectral Doppler w/ augment
6. SAG GSV: Calf
    a. P + M + D
        i. Color Doppler
        ii. Spectral Doppler w/ augment

Compress the GSV every 2cm, evaluating for clot

Upper Extremity

Patient Prep and Exam

The patient will need to remove their shirt. If the patient is wearing a bra and the strap gets in the way, I have them slide their arm out of the strap and have them tuck it under their arm and out of the way. We need to have access from the shoulder, down to the wrist.

Exam Indications

- Arterio-venous dialysis access

Normal Measurements

Structure:	Abbreviation/Acronym:	Measurements:
Cephalic	CEPH	>2.5mm
Basilic	BAS	>2.5mm

The measurements in the table above show the vessel AP requirements to be used as a dialysis shunt. Keep in mind that these superficial veins can become so small that they are not easily visible on US and that is normal.

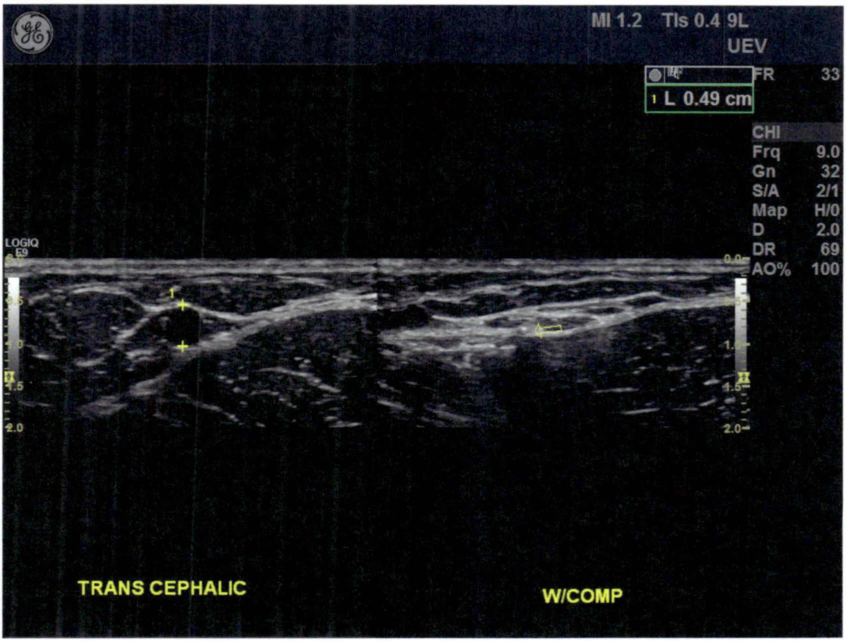

TRV cephalic vein with measurement on left and compressed / fully collapsed cephalic vein on right

Notes!

The first half of this protocol will be done in dual screen. The left side of the screen will be in TRV without compression, and the right side of the screen will be in TRV with compression. Take an AP measurement of the non-compressed vein on the left side of the screen. Document any and all evidence of obstruction. This again, refers to clot and intraluminal scarring.

Compress each vein every 2cm, evaluating for obstruction.

The second half of this protocol will be done in single-screen. We will evaluate the veins with both color and spectral Doppler.

Protocols

UE Vein Mapping

1. TRV CEPH V: Upper Arm
    a. P + M + D
        i. With and without compression + AP measurement of the non-compressed vein
2. TRV CEPH V: Forearm
    a. P + M + D
        i. With and without compression + AP measurement of the non-compressed vein
3. TRV BASIL V: Upper Arm
    a. P + M + D
        i. With and without compression + AP measurement of the non-compressed vein
4. TRV BASIL V: Forearm
    a. P + M + D
        i. With and without compression + AP measurement of the non-compressed vein
5. SAG CEPH V: Upper Arm
    a. P + M + D
        i. Color Doppler
        ii. Spectral Doppler w/ augment
6. SAG CEPH V: Forearm
    a. P + M + D
        i. Color Doppler
        ii. Spectral Doppler w/ augment
7. SAG BASIL V: Upper Arm
    a. P + M + D
        i. Color Doppler
        ii. Spectral Doppler w/ augment
8. SAG BASIL V: Forearm
    a. P + M + D
        i. Color Doppler
        ii. Spectral Doppler w/ augment

Compress the veins every 2cm, evaluating for clot

Notes

Notes

Notes

9

Appendix A

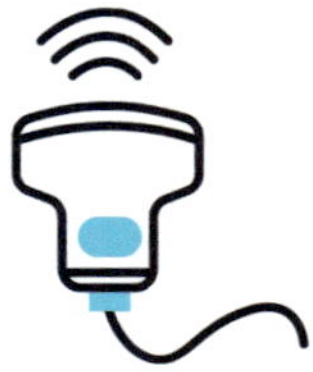

Navigating Bowel Gas

BOWEL GAS IS A common pitfall in ultrasound. It seems that nearly 100% of abdominal and pelvic exams will have bowel or bowel gas in the way of the organ we are evaluating. So, how do we get around it? Below are some tips and tricks on navigating this issue.

AORTA:

- Have the patient take a deep breath in and hold
- Scan lateral or medial to the bowel gas, then angle the transducer back towards the aorta
- Increase transducer pressure
- For the proximal aorta, scan using the intercostal approach. Use the liver

as a window and make sure to set the depth low enough to see the aorta. It's deeper than you think!

Pancreas:

- Scan superior to the pancreas in TRV, then angle the transducer down
- Have the patient take a deep breath in and hold
- Have the patient push / stick their stomach out, making it round

Kidneys:

- Roll the patient: LLD / RLD
- Have the patient take a deep breath in and hold
- Scan laterally along the patient's flank, superior to the hip
- For the right kidney, use the liver as a window
- Scan through the patient's back if all other techniques fail or if the patient is a child

Liver + Liver Vasculature + GB + CBD:

- Roll the patient: LLD
- Have the patient take a deep breath in and hold
- Use the intercostal spaces
- Have the patient raise their right arm over their head

Uterus + Ovaries + Prostate:

- Use the bladder as a window
- Increase transducer pressure
- Scan lateral or medial to the bowel gas, then angle the transducer back towards the organ

10

Appendix B

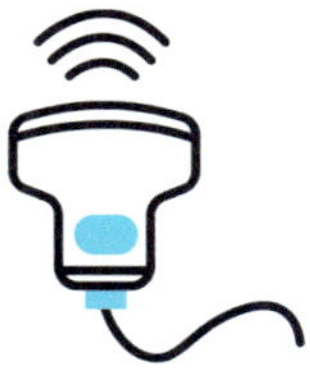

Pain

There are a few types of pain that we will commonly see in ultrasound. Let's discuss what those are.

Types of Pain

Acute Pain:

Pain that has a sudden onset and lasts anywhere from a couple of minutes to a couple of months. This pain typically subsides after healing or correcting the injury. This can occur from trauma or illness.

Examples:

- Broken bone

- Post-prandial pain
- Acute pancreatitis
- Cholecystitis
- Appendicitis

Chronic Pain:

Pain that has been occurring for 3+ months due to an injury or illness.

Examples:

- Chronic pancreatitis
- Arthritis
- Nerve damage
- Endometriosis
- IBS (Irritable Bowel Syndrome)

Post-Prandial Pain:

Pain that occurs in the abdomen after eating. This Most commonly occurs in the RUQ / epigastric region due to complications with the gallbladder.

Examples:

- Cholelithiasis
- Sludge

- Polyps
- GB perforation
- Cholecystitis

Ischemic Pain:

Pain due to blood flow reduction to the surrounding tissues. This can occur at rest (not during physical activity).

Symptoms:

- Cramping
- Aching
- Numbness
- Tingling

Claudication Pain:

Pain due to blood flow reduction to the surrounding tissues. This predominantly occurs during physical activity and improves with rest. This is a symptom of PAD (peripheral artery disease) and typically occurs in the buttocks and legs; such as, the calves.

Symptoms:

- Aching
- Cramping

- Pain
- Fatigue

Neuropathic Pain:

Pain that is caused from vascular diseases leading to poor circulation. This then leads to neuropathy (nerve damage).

Symptoms:

- Burning
- Tingling
- Sharp / shooting pain

Location of Pain

1. **Focal Pain:** Pain that is localized to one small area
2. **Global Pain:** Pain that is consistent across a vast majority of a structure or consumes the entire structure
3. **Referred Pain:** Pain that is felt in a different location from the actual source of pain
4. **Somatic Pain:** Pain that originates in the skin, muscles, and/or soft tissues
5. **Visceral Pain:** Pain that originates from internal organs

11

Appendix C

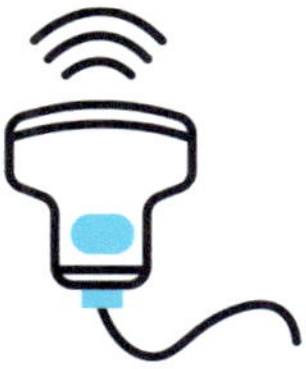

Patient Dignity

UPHOLDING PATIENT DIGNITY AND giving the best care is more than just being polite and scanning well. It's a dynamic set of things that when they come together, it provides the patient with an overall great experience. To give outstanding care to our patients we must be good at exhibiting a few key things.

Communication:

- Introducing yourself
- Explaining the exam you are performing and how long it will take
- Explaining how and when the patient will get results
- Answering questions they may have for clarification

Respect, Autonomy, and Choice:

- Letting the patient make decisions about their care
- Respecting the patient's decisions about their care
- Acknowledging the patient's feelings and concerns
- Recognizing their cultural background and how that reflects their beliefs and values

Privacy and Confidentiality:

- Asking patient identifying information questions and health related questions in the exam room and not in the hallways or commonly shared spaces with other patients and employees
- Keeping the patient as covered as possible for each exam, so they don't feel uncomfortable or too exposed

Comfort and Safety:

- Alleviating the patient of discomfort by offering the patient something such as a rolled up towel to help with neck pain, or a triangle pillow for under the knees for lower back pain
- Creating a safe environment by having access to wheelchairs, Hoyer lifts, other staff to help with transport, and security

Glossary

- **1st Trimester:** 0-13 weeks
- **2nd Trimester:** 14-27 weeks
- **3rd Trimester:** 28-40 weeks
- **Abdominal Circumference:** A fetal growth measurement taken around the abdomen. Landmarks for the image include the fetal stomach, umbilical vein, and portal sinus
- **Amniotic Fluid Index:** A quantitative measurement of the amniotic fluid in all four quadrants, calculating a total overall volume after 28 weeks gestational age only
- **Aneuploidy:** A chromosomal anomaly
- **Anhydramnios:** No amniotic fluid
- **Anteflexed:** A normal uterine anomaly where the uterus tilts upwards, and the fundus makes contact with the cervix
- **Anterior Placenta:** The placenta is located along the anterior wall of

the uterus

- **Anteverted:** A normal uterine anomaly where the uterus tilts upwards, however the fundus does not make contact with the cervix

- **Augment:** To squeeze distally to the area of the vein you are evaluating; forcing blood up the vein towards the heart. On spectral doppler you will see a dip in the waveform — that is the augment

- **BI-RADS:** Classification system to help determine what breast masses should be biopsied versus not

- **Biparietal Diameter:** A fetal growth measurement taken of the head. The landmarks for the image include the thalamus and CSP. This growth measurement is taken in the same image as the head circumference and is measured from outer anterior skull to inner posterior skull

- **Central Cord Insertion:** The cord inserts into the placenta centrally or in/near the middle

- **Cervical Funneling:** The premature opening of the internal os of the cervix, putting the fetus at risk for preterm birth

- **Claudication:** Pain, numbness, or fatigue in the legs while walking or standing, that is relieved during rest

- **Complete Placenta Previa:** The placenta completely covers the internal os of the cervix

- **Corpus Luteum:** The cyst that forms and ruptures within an ovary, releasing the egg. If the egg implants into the endometrium because fertilization occurs, the corpus luteum remains until the placenta forms, providing "nutrition" for the early gestation

- **Dichorionic — Diamniotic:** 2 chorions + 2 placentae, 2 amnions
- **Dilation and Curettage:** An invasive procedure done in the operating room. The cervix is dilated, and contents and/or portions of the endometrium are removed. This is a popular procedure for patients who have experienced a miscarriage in the 2nd trimester
- **Early Proliferative Phase:** Days 6-10 of the menstrual cycle
- **Fetal Breathing Movements:** The "act" of breathing is visualized in a fetus by the diaphragm contracting. This is evaluated and scored out of 2 on a BPP exam
- **Fetal Gross Movement:** Movements of the body. This is evaluated and scored out of 2 on a BPP exam
- **Fetal Tone:** The extension and flexion of the arms and legs. This is evaluated out of 2 on a BPP exam
- **Femur Length:** A fetal growth measurement taken of the femur bone
- **Focal Pain:** Pain that is localized to one small area
- **Fontanelle:** This is the soft spot on a baby's head. There are two on top of the head called the anterior and posterior fontanelles. The anterior fontanelle is the most commonly used for scanning the neonatal brain
- **Fundal Placenta:** The placenta is located within the uterine fundus
- **Glandular Tissue:** A collection of lobules and ducts in the breast that

produce milk and carry it to the nipple for breastfeeding

- **Global Pain:** Pain that is consistent across a vast majority of a structure or consumes the entire structure
- **Head Circumference:** A fetal growth measurement of the head. The landmarks for the image include the thalamus and CSP. This is taken in the same image as the biparietal diameter and is measured from outer anterior skull to outer posterior skull then using the ellipse tool, form the measurement to encase the entire head
- **Hepatofugal:** Blood flow away from the liver
- **Hepatopetal:** Blood flow towards the liver
- **Hyperemia/Hyperemic:** An increase in blood flow to an organ or location in the body
- **Intima-Media Thickness:** A measurement of the tunica intima and tunica media of a vessel
- **Intussusception:** The "telescoping" of bowel, causing bowel obstruction. *See the next two definitions for further elaboration*
- **Intussusceptum:** Prolapsed bowel that is pulled into the intussuscipiens
- **Intussuscipiens:** The bowel that receives the prolapsed bowel
- **Late Proliferative Phase:** Days 11-14 of the menstrual cycle
- **Lateral Cord Insertion:** The cord inserts into the placenta >2cm away from the placental edge

- **Left Lateral Decubitus:** The patient lies on their left side facing away from you
- **Low-lying Placenta:** The placenta is located within 2cm of the cervical internal os
- **Marginal Cord Insertion:** The cord inserts into the placenta within 2cm from the placental edge
- **Marginal Placenta Previa:** The placental tip just reaches the cervical internal os, but does not cover any portion of the cervix
- **Maximum Vertical Pocket:** Amniotic fluid assessment, but measuring the largest pocket (one of the four quadrants) in AP diameter
- **Menstrual Phase:** Days 1-5 of the menstrual cycle
- **Monochorionic — Diamnionic:** 1 chorion + placenta, 2 amnions
- **Monochorionic — Monoamniotic:** 1 chorion+ placenta, 1 amnion
- **Morison's Pouch:** The space between the liver and kidney. It can fill with blood or free fluid
- **Neonate:** A newborn infant
- **NPO:** *Nil per os*; meaning nothing to eat or drink by mouth
- **Nulliparous:** A woman who has never given birth
- **Oligohydramnios**: Too little amniotic fluid
- **Parous:** A woman who has given birth at least once
- **Partial Placenta Previa:** The placenta covers a portion of the cervical

internal os

- **PO:** Per os; meaning by mouth
- **Polyhydramnios:** Too much amniotic fluid
- **Posterior Placenta:** The placenta is located along the posterior wall of the uterus
- **Prone:** The patient lies face down – on their abdomen
- **Rebound Tenderness:** Pain is induced when pressure from a hand or object (such as a transducer) is removed
- **Referred Pain:** Pain that is felt in a different location from the actual source of pain
- **Retroflexed:** A normal uterine anomaly where the uterus tilts backward, and the fundus makes contact with the cervix
- **Retroverted:** A normal uterine anomaly where the uterus tilts backward, however the fundus does not make contact with the cervix
- **Right Lateral Decubitus:** The patient lies on their right side facing toward you
- **Right/Left Lateral Lying Placenta:** The placenta is located either to the right or left in the uterus. It will also be either anterior or posterior in location
- **Secretory Phase:** Days 15-28 of the menstrual cycle
- **Somatic Pain:** Pain that originates in the skin, muscles, and/or soft tissues

- **Splenomegaly:** An enlarged spleen
- **TI-RADS:** Classification system to help determine what thyroid nodules should be biopsied versus not
- **TIPS:** A shunt that is connected from the portal vein to a hepatic vein. This shunt helps bypass blood that would otherwise flow through the liver. This helps patients that suffer from portal hypertension in cases of liver failure by reducing the pressure in the portal vein
- **Velamentous Cord Insertion:** The cord inserts into the chorio-amniotic membranes, then travels between them (chorion + amnion) to the placenta
- **Visceral Pain:** Pain that originates from internal organs

Acknowledgements

I have so many people to thank because it took quite a large team to assemble this book from the editors to the volunteer models.

A big thank you to my fellow coworkers and radiologists that have helped me look over my work. Without you guys, there would be no way that this book would look as polished. From the precise editing to the detailed overview of the measurements. I can't tell you how much I appreciate every single one of you for helping me with this project. I am truly grateful. To name just a few;

Thank you Jed Peterson, MD for taking the time and being so gracious to give me your notes and edits. I really appreciate your help with my book and helping make it informative and up to date with the latest information.

Another thank you to Yuliya Walters RT (R) (M) (BD) for looking over and editing my breast chapter, as well as, being a model. It is such a privilege to have a coworker like you. I appreciate your expertise in the mammography field and helping out with my book. You are one of the sweetest people I know and I love working with you!

Thank you to Matthew Huff, RVT for taking the time to read through and edit my vascular chapter. I really appreciate your time and kindness with your feedback. You have truly helped shape this chapter of my book by helping provide the most accurate information out there today. Thank you for what you do!

Thank you to my models for letting me take images of their anatomy to share with all of you! Thank you to Kara B. CPT, Robert Mulder RT (R), Andrea VanHuizen Brewer RT (R) (M), Sydney Stearns RT (R), Elena Yasinskiy, and all of my other models. I really appreciate you all for coming in and letting me take images. Without you, this book wouldn't be anywhere near as good!

A special thanks to UltrasoundCases.info and SonoSkills.com for generously permitting the use of their pyloric stenosis and intussusception images for my pediatric abdomen chapter. Those images added valuable information and I thank you for helping make these details more accessible. Without those images, it would be harder to grasp the ultrasound presentation of each condition.

I am so thankful for my entire family. To name just a few, thank you to my mom, dad, yiayia, and papoo. I am very lucky to have such a wonderful support system at home. You all encourage me everyday to strive after my goals and to not give up. Thank you for always listening to me and giving me feedback when I talk non-stop about all of my book projects. I love you all very much.

References

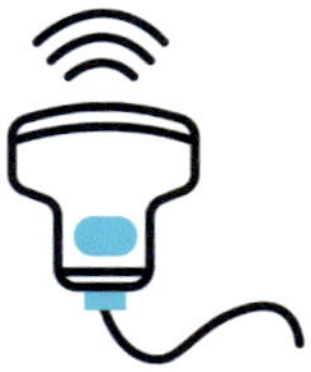

Amini, Behrang. "Pyloric Stenosis | Radiology Reference Article | Radiopaedia.org." *Radiopaedia*, 2 May 2008, radiopaedia.org/articles/pyloric-stenosis-1?lang=us.
Last revision on Dec. 22, 2024.

Columbia Surgery. "The Pancreas and Its Functions." *Columbia Surgery*, Oct. 2024, columbiasurgery.org/pancreas/pancreas-and-its-functions.

Curry, PhD, RT(R), RDMS, Reva Arnez, and Betty Bates Tempkin, BA. *Sonography: Introduction to Normal Structure and Function*. 4th ed., Elsevier, 2016, pp. 141–155, 158, 172, 181–182, 227, 229, 233, 265, 267, 271, 294–298, 306, 334, 340, 342, 391, 410, 446, 494, 497–498, 518.

Dighe, Manjiri, et al. "NEONATAL HIP ULTRASOUND PROTOCOL for DEVELOPMENTAL DYSPLASIA." 15 Jan. 2023.

Gaillard, Frank. "Developmental Dysplasia of the Hip | Radiology Reference Article | Radiopaedia.org." *Radiopaedia.org*, 2 May 2008, radiopaedia.org/articles/developmental-dysplasia-of-the-hip.
Last revised on Jan. 8, 2025.

---. "Gallbladder | Radiology Reference Article | Radiopaedia.org." *Radiopaedia*, 22 Nov. 2010, radiopaedia.org/articles/gallbladder.
Last revision on Feb. 10, 2025 by Arlene Campos.

Gornik, Heather L, et al. *ACCF/ACR/AIUM/ASE/IAC/SCAI/SCVS/SIR/SVM/SVS/SVU 2013 Appropriate Use Criteria for Peripheral Vascular Ultrasound and Physiological Testing Part II: Testing for Venous Disease and Evaluation of Hemodialysis Access*. Vol. 62, no. 7, 1 Aug. 2013, pp. 649–665, www.jacc.org/doi/10.1016/j.jacc.2013.05.001#sec10.1, https://doi.org/10.1016/j.jacc.2013.05.001. Accessed 28 June 2023.

Hagen-Ansert, MS, RDMS, RDCS, FASE, FSDMS, Sandra L. *Textbook of Diagnostic Sonography*. 8th ed., vol. 2, Elsevier, 2018, pp. 1056, 1059, 1061, 1188.

---. *Textbook of Diagnostic Sonography* . 8th ed., vol. 1, Elsevier, 2018, pp. 145, 202, 249–250, 285, 376, 619, 634, 643.

Hall, Rebecca. *The Ultrasound Handbook*. 1993. 3rd ed., Lippincott Williams & Wilkins, 1999, pp. 1, 135, 211, 223, 236.

Henry Suarez. "Neonatal Neurosonography." *Sonographic Tendencies*, 7 Nov. 2016, sonographictendencies.com/2016/11/07/neonatal-neursonography/.

Johns Hopkins Medicine. "Liver: Anatomy and Functions." *Johns Hopkins Medicine*, www.hopkinsmedicine.org/health/conditions-and-diseases/liver-anatomy-and-functions.

Jones, Jeremy, and Frank Gaillard. "Nuchal Translucency." *Radiopaedia.org*, 2 May 2008, https://doi.org/10.53347/rid-1742.
Revised on Jan. 17, 2025.

Jones, Jeremy, and Yaïr Glick. "Head Ultrasound." *Radiopaedia.org*, 26 Jan. 2020, https://doi.org/10.53347/rid-73886.

Jones, Jeremy, and Matt Morgan. "Bladder Wall Thickening (Differential)." *Radiopaedia.org*, 8 Dec. 2014, https://doi.org/10.53347/rid-32648.
Last revised on Aug. 6, 2024.

Jones, Jeremy, and Yuranga Weerakkody. "Variation in Cord Insertion." *Radiopaedia.org*, 13 Apr. 2011, https://doi.org/10.53347/rid-13466.
Last revised on Spet. 20, 2021.

Kecler-Pietrzyk, Aneta. "Normal Kidney Size in Adults | Radiology Reference Article | Radiopaedia.org." *Radiopaedia*, 29 Apr. 2017, radiopaedia.org/articles/normal-kidney-size-in-adults?lang=us.
Last revised on Jan 19, 2023 by Cilein Kearns.

Maingard, Julian. "Prostate | Radiology Reference Article | Radiopaedia.org." *Radiopaedia.org*, 25 Nov. 2013, radiopaedia.org/articles/prostate. Last revision on Oct. 10, 2024 by Craig Hacking.

Marion, Becky. "Neonatal Cranial Ultrasound Protocol NEONATAL CRANIAL ULTRASOUND PROTOCOL (UENC)." 1 June 2022.

Mohler, Emile R., et al. "ACCF/ACR/AIUM/ASE/ASN/ICAVL/SCAI/SCCT/SIR/SVM/SVS 2012 Appropriate Use Criteria for Peripheral Vascular Ultrasound and Physiological Testing Part I: Arterial Ultrasound and Physiological Testing." *Journal of the American College of Cardiology*, vol. 60, no. 3, July 2012, pp. 242–276, pmc.ncbi.nlm.nih.gov/articles/PMC4634367/#S7, https://doi.org/10.1016/j.jacc.2012.02.009. Accessed 7 Apr. 2022.

"Neonatal Spine Normal – ULTRASOUNDPAEDIA." *Ultrasoundpaedia*, ultrasoundpaedia.com/neonatal-spine-normal/.

Ozturk, Arinc, et al. "PRINCIPLES of ULTRASOUND ELASTOGRAPHY." *Abdominal Radiology (New York)*, vol. 43, no. 4, 1 Apr. 2018, pp. 773–785, www.ncbi.nlm.nih.gov/pmc/articles/PMC5973820/, https://doi.org/10.1007/s00261-018-1475-6.

"Pancreas Normal." *Ultrasoundpaedia*, ultrasoundpaedia.com/pancreas-normal/.

Pellerito, MD, FACR, FSRU, FAIUM, John S., and Joseph F. Polak, MD, MPH. *Introduction to Vascular Sonography*. 6th ed., Elsevier Saunders, 2012, pp. 136–140, 163, 194–195, 25–252, 298, 450, 486, 498, 523.

Radiology Video. "Ultrasound Liver Elastography." *YouTube*, 19 Dec. 2018, www.youtube.com/watch?v=GCBTnJW-Hzw. Accessed 19 July 2021. Speaker: Richard G. Barr, MD, PhD.

Radquarters. "Ultrasound of Intussusception." *YouTube*, 25 May 2023, www.youtube.com/watch?v=O6ZjG9c_b-I. Speaker: Daniel J. Kowal, MD.

Robben, Simon, and Robin Smithuis. "The Radiology Assistant: Developmental Dysplasia of the Hip Ultrasound Examination." *Radiology Assistant*, 1 Dec. 2017, radiologyassistant.nl/pediatrics/hip/developmental-dysplasia-of-the-hip-ultrasound.

Rumack, M.D., Carol M. , et al. *Diagnostic Ultrasound* . 3rd ed., Elsevier Mosby, 2005, pp. 82, 149, 172–173, 214, 322, 532, 554, 737, 849.

Siegel, Marilyn J. *Pediatric Sonography*. 4th ed., Lippincott Williams & Wilkins, a Wolters Kluwer Business, 2011, pp. 43–60, 65, 605, 647–654.

Sonography Student Studies. "Liver Elastography." *YouTube*, 27 Jan. 2022, www.youtube.com/watch?v=bkzYUZ3CStg. Accessed 9 Dec. 2024.

"Sonoguide // Gallbladder." *American College of Emergency Physicians*, 10 June 2020, www.acep.org/sonoguide/basic/gallbladder/.

SonoSkills.com, and UltrasoundCases.Info. *Hypertrophic Pyloric Stenosis*, www.ultrasoundcases.info/hypertrophic-pyloric-stenosis-2028/. Accessed 7 June 2025.

SonoSkills.com, and UltrasoundCases.info. *Target Shaped Lesion in the Left Upper Abdomen*, Mar. 2009, www.ultrasoundcases.info/march-2009-4568/. Accessed 9 July 2025.

"Spleen Normal – ULTRASOUNDPAEDIA." *Radiopaedia*, ultrasoundpaedia.com/spleen-normal/.

Suarez, Henry . "Pyloric Ultrasound." *Sonographic Tendencies*, 16 Nov. 2016, sonographictendencies.com/2016/11/16/pyloric-ultrasound/.

Weerakkody, Yuranga. "Hepatic Arterial Resistive Index." *Radiopaedia*, Radiopaedia.org, 12 May 2010, radiopaedia.org/articles/hepatic-arterial-resistive-index.
Last revised on March 23, 2023.

---. "Pancreatic Duct Diameter | Radiology Reference Article | Radiopaedia.org." *Radiopaedia*, 1 Sept. 2013, radiopaedia.org/articles/pancreatic-duct-diameter.
Last revision on Feb. 26, 2024.

---. "Velamentous Cord Insertion | Radiology Reference Article | Radiopaedia.org." *Radiopaedia*, 13 Apr. 2011, radiopaedia.org/articles/velamentous-cord-insertion?lang=us.
Last revised on Aug. 20, 2024.

Wei Oh, Chia. "Common Bile Duct | Radiology Reference Article | Radiopaedia.org." *Radiopaedia*, 14 Sept. 2013, radiopaedia.org/articles/common-bile-duct-2?lang=us.
Last revised on July 5, 2024 by Tariq Walizai.

Weill, F, et al. "Ultrasonography of the Normal Pancreas." *Radiology*, vol. 123, no. 2, 1 May 1977, pp. 417–423, pubs.rsna.org/doi/abs/10.1148/123.2.417, https://doi.org/10.1148/123.2.417.

Woodward, MD, Paula J. , et al. *Diagnostic Imaging Obstetrics*. 3rd ed., Elsevier, 2016, pp. 72–86, 232–235.

Zwiebel, MD, William J., and John S. Pellerito, MD. *Introduction to Vascular Ultrasonography*. 5th ed., Elsevier Saunders, 2005, pp. 306, 330–331, 346.

Also by the Author

Ultrasound:

A Guide for Prospective Students on Becoming a Sonographer

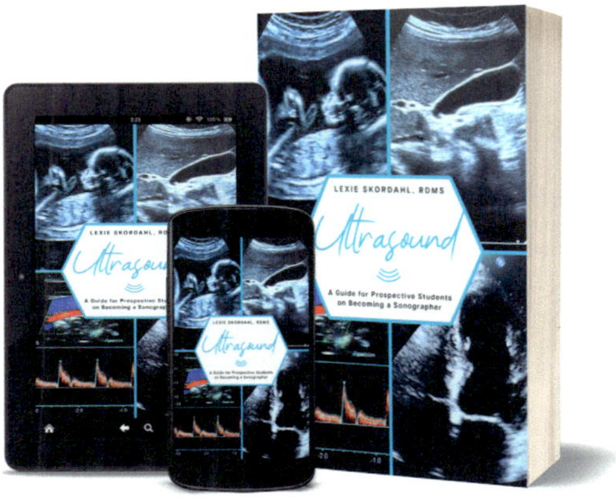

Available on Amazon and Barnes & Noble

This guide is for those who wish to become a sonographer and want a more in-depth look at what being a sonographer really entails.

Note From the Author

Hey guys! I hope this guide was a helpful quick reference for you and your team. We have to memorize so many things in our field and I know it can be easy to forget things if you haven't looked at them in a while, hence why I wanted to create this guide.

If you were hoping that I covered something a little bit more in-depth or if you still have a question that was left unanswered, please feel free to reach me at sonographerlexie@gmail.com. I will try my best to respond in a timely manner.

If you enjoyed this guide, please leave a review and spread the word to your friends and coworkers. That would be very much appreciated!

Find Me On Social Media!

TikTok: @lexieskordahlauthor

Instagram: @sonographer_lexie

Facebook: Sonographer Lexie

About the Author

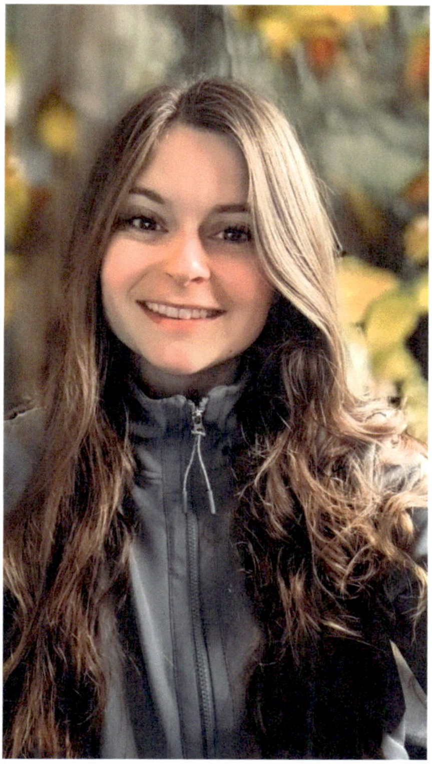

Lexie is an ARDMS registered sonographer in AB, OB/GYN, RVT, and BR. She completed her schooling in Washington state, interned at a hospital in Bellevue WA and a clinic in Vancouver WA. She now works at a fantastic hospital near her hometown. She loves speaking and teaching to prospective and current students and is always happy to share her knowledge and love of ultrasound with others.

Made in the USA
Las Vegas, NV
03 November 2026

57424839R00181